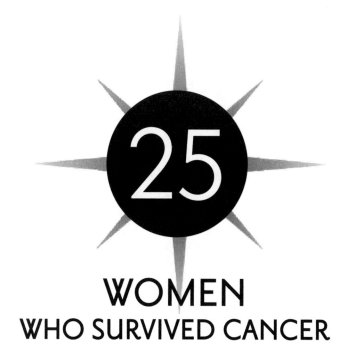

WOMEN
WHO SURVIVED CANCER

NOTABLE WOMEN SHARE INSPIRING STORIES OF HOPE

KT-376-819

Edited by Mark Evan Chimsky

SELLERS
PUBLISHING

Contents

Preface

As the American Cancer Society reminds us, everyone is affected by cancer in one way or another. I was directly affected when one of the senior staff members of the publishing company I own came into my office and told me she'd been diagnosed with breast cancer. I had worked closely with this woman for many years, so of course the news was upsetting to me on many levels. Despite my assurances that we would figure out a way to cover for her while she was undergoing treatment, she insisted that she wanted to continue coming in to work and guaranteed me that she would uphold her responsibilities as much as possible while working to cure herself of her cancer.

During the years that followed, I was amazed by this woman's courage and strength of character. I was also humbled by her dedication to her job and the people she supervised. Throughout her treatment process she kept me apprised of how she was progressing. Then, on a day I will never forget, she came in and said exuberantly, "I'm about to pass my five-year anniversary. I've been cancer-free for five years!" She explained that this was an important milestone for women being treated for breast cancer. Once passing that five-year mark, the odds of staying in remission increase dramatically. Needless to say, this was very happy news!

As a result of this experience, I began thinking about creating a book that would offer people dealing with cancer hope and inspiration. Many book publishers are reluctant to publish books on the subject of cancer. I can't tell you how many publishing colleagues have said to me, "Cancer, now THAT'S a tough subject. Nobody wants to read books about cancer."

"Except for people who are dealing with cancer," was always my reply. I knew from my own experience that there are many, many people who have been treated and cured of their cancer. That's good news, especially if you are undergoing treatment yourself. I realized a great approach would be to reach out to women who had been diagnosed with cancer, undergone treatment, and survived, and to ask them to write about their experiences.

I contacted Mark Chimsky, a highly respected and experienced editor whom I trust implicitly, and asked him if he would be interested in assuming responsibility for compiling and editing 25 Women Who Survived Cancer.

PREFACE

Mark loved the idea and immediately agreed to take on the project.

Mark was relentless when it came to reaching out to well-known cancer survivors for written contributions to this book. He did a fabulous job. The list of contributors speaks for itself, and I will be forever grateful for his professionalism and enthusiasm during the editorial process.

I am even more grateful to the women who valued this project enough to contribute their wonderfully stirring essays, all of which are on a subject that is deeply personal. Just as it takes courage to fight cancer, it takes courage to share the details of the experience. Their stories are powerful, informational, emotional, and often (believe it or not) funny in a most human way. Most importantly, they are real. And therein lies the power of this book. It is a collection of real stories about real women who faced cancer, fought cancer, and won. It is a testament to the power of hope. Could there be anything more inspiring than that?

Ronnie Sellers
President & Publisher
Sellers Publishing, Inc.

Introduction

In 25 Women Who Survived Cancer, you will find inspiring essays by notable women of a diverse range of ages, backgrounds, and perspectives, writing about their personal experiences with a wide spectrum of cancers, including breast cancer; uterine, cervical, and ovarian cancer; Hodgkin lymphoma; and malignant melanoma. While going through the editing process, I noticed a number of common themes running through the essays. In one way or another, many of the contributors start out by acknowledging that "cancer sucks." That's to be expected. What is constantly surprising — and compelling — is how the perspective pivots to a new insight: that because of cancer, they have become stronger, and more in touch with who they are as they forge deep connections with others. The contributors don't *tell* us they're heroes — but we are *shown* examples of their courage in the stories they share. We see the extraordinary transformations that occur as they move from anger to acceptance, from resistance to realization, from fear to joy. In each essay, there are examples of bravery in action as well as revelations about the kinds of ordinary miracles that help to turn obstacles into opportunities.

All these essays have gifts to offer, whether it's Robin Roberts writing about going public with her baldness as a way of "reaching out to others who had faced cancer"; or Joan Lunden listing the six things that medical professionals need to know — and do — to treat cancer patients more effectively and humanely; or Liz Lange charting the steps that helped her beat cervical cancer and discussing how she decided to tell her story "to as many media outlets as possible in the hopes of making sure that all women saw their health-care providers regularly."

Each personal essay in the book strikes a memorable chord. Among them are: Barbara Musser at a clothing-optional "Love, Intimacy, and Sexuality" workshop after healing from cancer surgery, standing naked and vulnerable in front of everyone in attendance, and feeling the waves of love and acceptance; Caryn Hartglass seeing the cosmic connection between a famous painting and her own cancer experience; Marissa Jaret Winokur writing of how she wouldn't let her radical hysterectomy stand in the way of her dream of becoming a mom.

In addition to the twenty-five essays in this book, there is a bonus essay, written by a survivor of another kind. Fifteen-year-old Capri Ruberto Anderson was on the front lines watching her mother Nina go through the difficulties of her cancer diagnosis and treatment. At twelve, Capri wanted to show her love for her mom, so she used her musical talent to write Nina a song called "Hope." Capri's performance of the song went viral and captured the hearts of many. I am honored that Nina's powerful account of surviving cancer is followed by Capri's beautiful essay that emphasizes, and exemplifies, the importance of support of families and friends.

Perhaps one of the most poignant images that emerges in this collection occurs in the essay by Pamela Rafalow Grossman. Pamela uses the metaphor of "Cancer Island" to convey how disoriented she felt when she was first diagnosed. Gradually, however, she discovers that Cancer Island "offers great company." Like so many of her fellow contributors, Pamela acknowledges her cancer experiences but refuses to let them consume her identity. "A cancer diagnosis may be a part of someone's life," she writes, "but it does not define that life, and it never will."

In many of these heartfelt essays, the contributors write with exceptional candor about how their experiences have given them a new sense of purpose. As Nina Ruberto says, "I have never felt so ALIVE." We see it manifest in how these survivors now live their lives, speaking up for themselves and speaking out as advocates to raise awareness about cancer, and pursuing their dreams — whether it's Dr. Ruth Heidrich, who at eighty years old is a "breast-cancer-thriver triathlete" or Sylvia McNair, who feels blessed to have the opportunity to "sing [her] Truth." Joanna Laufer sees comfort and hope in the lesson "that every fear and challenge we faced will strengthen, heal, and free us."

Each essay describes a personal journey, often internal but also external as well. Rachael Yahne, who was diagnosed with cancer at seventeen, writes eloquently of her trip to Greece to "commemorate a decade of survivorship." As she reflects back on what cancer took from her, she also honors what the experience has given her. With keen insight, she reveals that the lesson that cancer teaches is not only about fighting — but also about forgiving and being grateful: "Forgiveness is waiting just inside our hearts, but our own fears and wants keep us from reaching out for its hand and climbing to the other side. But when we stop keeping track of what's fair and what's not, and stop asking life to give as much as we give, we can take a look around at all we really have."

Editing this book became an amazing learning process for me. I am grateful to the contributors for tapping into experiences that were painful, holding nothing back as they describe the moments when they first received their diagnosis, or started their treatments, or were given the news that there was no longer any evidence of disease.

It was a privilege to be allowed inside their world, where each contributor generously shared stories of pain, but also of transformation. They teach how to deal with the unexpected — to fight with astonishing reserves, to become one's own strongest advocate, and to see that even in adversity we can learn something of value that helps us grow.

I was struck over and over by how their stories resonate with hard-won truths and hope. The personal truly is universal. A number of the contributors have told me how difficult it was to relive certain experiences in order to write about them, how they had to struggle to go deep into a past that they would simply prefer to forget. But they went to those hard places and they took those painful journeys because they felt it would do others some good. That is the spirit that has guided this project from the beginning.

It is therefore my hope that you will find stories in these pages that will speak directly to you and give you strength to move on. The women in this book are paying it forward, giving something of themselves to all of us who read their essays.

I am grateful to Ronnie Sellers for coming up with the idea for this project and for giving me the opportunity to put it all together. I am also indebted to Robin Haywood for her support and feedback as this book took shape.

Now, at the end of the months of compiling and editing these essays, what I have discovered, to my own surprise, is that 25 Women Who Survived Cancer is ultimately a celebration. Of life. Of renewal. Of liberation. Of gratitude. As Jennifer Hayden writes in an excerpt from her funny, moving graphic memoir, The Story of My Tits, "All you can do is celebrate making it through. And give the damage its due." And this is the way Barbara Delinsky exuberantly defines it: "Suddenly, formally, I was a survivor. In common parlance, that means I've been diagnosed with breast cancer and am still alive. But, wait. *Still alive?* Is that all? Hell, no. For me, it wasn't about being *still alive* but about having my life suddenly, richly, *lushly* open wide before me! That's what *liberated* means." She sees this and every future shift in thinking about being a survivor as "a cause for celebration."

May each of you who reads this book find your own truth reflected in the truths expressed in these essays. May each of you draw courage from the courageous stories of this sisterhood of survivors. As you read this book, take to heart the words of Capri Ruberto Anderson's song for her mother, "Hope is by our side."

Mark Evan Chimsky

May 2016

ROBIN ROBERTS is the anchor of ABC's morning show *Good Morning America*. Under her leadership, the broadcast has won three consecutive Emmy Awards for Outstanding Morning Program. Prior to that, Robin was a contributor to ESPN. She is a native of Mississippi Gulf Coast and currently resides in New York City.

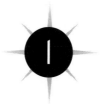

Everybody's Got Something

Robin Roberts
with Veronica Chambers

After *GMA* [in the] morning, I flew to Atlanta for an assignment. As the plane pulled up to the gate, I turned on my BlackBerry and cell phone. There was an e-mail from my then assistant, Ayana, saying that Dr. Knapp's office had called, and I needed to answer my cell phone because he would be trying to reach me. Just as I finished reading Ayana's message, my phone rang. It was Dr. Knapp. He asked if there was any way I could come to his office. I told him I was on the road and to please just give me the news now. He didn't want to but I insisted. I was still in my seat on the plane when he gave me the test results. "Robin, it's cancer."

I know he said more than that, but to me it sounded like the adults talking in a *Peanuts* cartoon. "Wawpp, wawpp, wawpp . . . CANCER . . . wawpp, wawpp, wawpp." I do recall agreeing to have a breast MRI the next day in New York and to meet with a breast surgeon.

There is no way to prepare yourself to hear the words: *You have cancer.* Trust me, it's less than ideal to be sitting on a plane when you hear it. After all, in the movies when you learn you have cancer you're seated in the doctor's office holding a loved one's hand. I was all by myself, surrounded by strangers, about to get off a plane in Atlanta. When I boarded in New York I was just Robin. Now I was Robin with breast cancer. My eyes started to fill with tears, and I put on sunglasses so no one would notice.

A driver was waiting to take me to Pine Mountain, Georgia. I wanted to call Amber. We'd been dating less than two years at that point. I also wanted to call my family and friends to let them know I had cancer. But I didn't want the driver to know what was going on, because I wasn't ready for the public to learn about my diagnosis. I'd only had minutes to digest it myself. The driver could not have been nicer, but he was also a bit inquisitive, and I knew he'd be listening in on my conversation. So I played a little guessing game with my loved ones. "Remember how I told you I was going to have that thing checked out?" I asked, in a quivering voice. "What do you think I found out?" I guess my tone was a dead giveaway. They knew. They'd been praying for the best, but were prepared for the worst. And here it was. The Big C.

Revealing my diagnosis to Amber and my family was difficult. I remember in particular telling Sally-Ann. She was just back in her flood-damaged home that had taken nearly two years to rebuild following Hurricane Katrina. I called Sally-Ann and she sounded so happy. She was in her car at the drive-thru of the newly rebuilt Popeye's near her neighborhood in New Orleans. (We both like two pieces of white meat — spicy — with french fries.) When I told Sally-Ann I had bad news she got out of line and parked her car. Then I took a deep breath and I told my oldest sister that I had been diagnosed with breast cancer. Willie, her college sweetheart and husband of twenty-five years, had died of colon cancer the day before Thanksgiving in 2002. I could hear the fear in her voice that she could lose me, too.

What is so remarkable about that day is that in the midst of being scared and shaking with my personal crisis, I could become so uplifted and inspired by bearing witness to someone else's tragedy. As my mom always said, everybody's got something. I was in Pine Mountain to interview Michael and Jeri Bishop, whose only son, Jamie, had been killed a few months earlier in the horrific shootings that took place at Virginia Tech in 2007. Jamie had been a beloved teacher there, and his parents were still numb with grief. Nevertheless, they had agreed to talk to me for a story that would air the first day the students returned to campus in Blacksburg.

The Bishops are such lovely people. They welcomed me into their home and fed me delicious cherries. Their warmth touched me, and it was all I could do not to collapse into their arms and cry, "I have cancer." But I pulled myself together. They had lost their son in one of the most tragic ways imaginable. I was there to comfort them.

The Bishops spoke so eloquently and movingly about Jamie. When I asked them what they wanted the students returning to know, Jeri said, "I want them to know that they are in the right place at the right time." Her comment was in reference to President George W. Bush's words during a memorial service that the thirty-two people killed were in the wrong place at the wrong time. The Bishops felt that despite the tragedy, their incredible son had been where he was supposed to be. He was a passionate teacher making a difference in countless lives.

I hugged the Bishops good-bye and got back in the car to return to the airport. I was desperate for some privacy. All I wanted was to get home. But wouldn't you know it, my flight was delayed, and it was almost 11 p.m. before I walked through my front door. I crumbled like an accordion on my couch and had a good long cry. Something I had wanted to do ever since I heard Dr. Knapp utter those words almost twelve hours earlier.

The next day I had a breast MRI, and Amber went with me to meet my surgeon, Lauren Cassell. She's the absolute best: a little dynamo in designer dresses and killer high heels, a force of nature, adored by all her patients. Dr. Cassell clearly explained the situation to me. My tumor appeared to be a little more than two centimeters. During surgery she would also check my lymph nodes. I barely have a scar thanks to her brilliant work. More important, she expertly removed my tumor and got clean margins the first time. She spends countless hours reviewing X-rays and images of the breast. She's gifted in knowing how much beyond the tumor to remove. Cancerous tumors are tricky, because it's not just removing the tumor but also any minute particles it may leave behind. Many patients have to go back a second or third time because the surgeon didn't get enough. Not the case with Lauren Cassell.

I endured many months of chemotherapy and radiation. I remember when my hair started to fall out from the chemo. My beloved mother was staying with me. She wanted to be with her baby girl when I began treatment. Two weeks after my first dose of chemo my hair started coming out in clumps. Momma was in my kitchen cooking her world-famous collard greens. I went to her bawling my eyes out, holding chunks of my hair. She sweetly comforted me with one arm, while stirring her collards with the other. I don't think she wanted me to get too close to her pot of delicious greens. I cherish that memory.

Amber, my dear siblings and friends were there for me every step of the way. Diane Sawyer was a constant source of comfort. We always have each other's backs. In fact, to celebrate my last chemo treatment, Diane snuck in some Popeye's chicken for me — she has a knack for knowing exactly what you want. Diane also knew my mind was always racing and so I had a hard time sleeping. She would send me a message late at night and tell me: "You can get some rest, I'll take it from here, I'm on watch now."

My emotions were all over the map. I was scared, angry, confused and even embarrassed. Yes, I said "embarrassed." How could I have cancer? I prided myself on being health conscious and athletic. Would people think I had done something wrong? Did I think I had done something wrong? A million questions raced through my bewildered mind, and none of them had answers.

Later answers did come, and the most lasting one came from my mother, who urged me to use my diagnosis to raise awareness about the importance of mammograms and early detection. "Make your mess your message," Momma liked to say. And I did.

The video diary that I made of my hairstylist, Petula, shaving my head after chemo started causing my hair to fall out in clumps touched millions of viewers. I had worn a wig on *GMA*, because I didn't want my *baldness* to distract from the stories I was covering. *People* magazine was about to publish a story about my battle with cancer. The article would include never-before-seen pictures of me bald. I didn't want *GMA* viewers to think I had been keeping something from them, that I was ashamed of my bald head. Instead I felt that my baldness and all it represented could become an important part of the story — another way of reaching out to others who had faced cancer. Do you know that some women actually refuse to be treated for fear of losing their hair? In the words of my friend India Arie: "Hey, I am not my hair. I am not this skin. I am a soul that lives within." I wanted to make a statement that I wasn't ashamed to have cancer or be bald. I was absolutely stunned by the reaction to my video diary. The outpouring of support was overwhelming.

Not long after my video diary, I ran into a woman at Bitz-n-Pieces; it's a wig store in New York. It's really much more than that. The talented people who work there are like little angels. Many clients are there looking for answers at difficult times in their lives.

This particular woman and I were bringing our wigs in for tune-ups. She said I had given her the strength to talk to her friends and her colleagues about her illness. I was thrilled for her, because I knew she was now opening herself up to a source of great comfort. She said she had hidden her illness from them for fear that they would treat her differently. But her friends had seen that I was still able to work, and that gave her the courage to speak openly.

Midway through my treatments, I was at the White House to do an interview with President Bush's press secretary, Tony Snow. He had recently revealed he was facing cancer for a second time. While there I was told that the First Lady, Laura Bush, wanted to see me in the private residence for tea. Mrs. Bush has a family history of breast cancer. She personally invited me to accompany her on a portion of an international breast cancer initiative with the Susan G. Komen Foundation, and I couldn't pass up this opportunity. My doctors cleared me to travel — although getting my mom's blessing was far more difficult. Remember, I was in the middle of chemo treatments. I spent time with Mrs. Bush in Abu Dhabi and Dubai, in the UAE and in Riyadh, Saudi Arabia. I met some incredible women on the trip. Breast cancer is the number one killer of women in the UAE. Many succumb because the stigma surrounding the disease in that part of the world prevents them from seeking early detection.

Cancer forced me out of my comfort zone. But the reality is that in life, there are no true comfort zones. Life comes at us in ways that we can't predict or control. My breast cancer battle taught me that, more than almost any other challenge I had faced to date. By the time I was cancer-free, I was confident that I'd gotten the lessons and I'd done the work that had been my spiritual assignment. Cancer was nothing more than a chapter in my life's story. It would never *be* my life's story.

At the same time, I made a very personal decision. I decided, and I let my closest friends know, that if I got cancer a second time, I would not seek treatment. I would roll the dice and live as long as I could, on my own terms.

I'd just had a grueling chemo treatment, the type of chemo that was nicknamed "the Red Devil" because of its color. I wanted to crush the syringe with my bare hands. I felt the worst I had ever felt at that point.

During that treatment, I was literally on my knees, looking up at the heavens and whispering, "Oh God, no more. No more. Not again. No *mas*."

I honestly thought I wouldn't put myself through this ever again. No more poison coursing through my veins. No more tubes. No more needles. I thought, "I'll take the time I have left and I will travel the world." Maybe I'd finally get my pilot's license. But no more barbaric treatments that tortured my body with only a vague promise to prolong my life. What kind of life would that be?

But this is the thing. Everything changed when I was diagnosed with MDS. The doctors said that a transplant would not be treatment, but a cure. I knew that there was a cure on the table. Even though it meant more chemo, even though I knew that my immune system would be destroyed and then rebuilt again, cell by cell, I had only one thought: "I want to live."

CARYN HARTGLASS holds Bachelor and Master of Science degrees in Chemical Engineering from Bucknell University. She recently obtained the Plant-Based Nutrition Certificate from eCornell and T. Colin Campbell Center for Nutrition Studies, and the Food Protection Certificate from the New York City Department of Health and Mental Hygiene. Caryn is passionate about helping people understand the effects of food choices on health and environment. She is the co-founder of the nonprofit organization Responsible Eating And Living (REAL), which delivers easy-to-use, factual information and services, providing inspiration to help each one of us take responsibility to nourish, protect, and support ourselves, our families, and the Earth with whole, plant-based foods and planet-friendly products. Caryn is also the co-director of the online nutrition, health, and wellness programs at the Food Revolution Network with Ocean and John Robbins. Prior to REAL, Caryn was the Executive Director of EarthSave International. An ovarian cancer survivor, Caryn combines science with practical knowledge from real-life experiences lecturing around the world about the powerful, healing benefits of a plant-based diet, juicing, and meditation. She has appeared on the *Dr. Oz Show, Geraldo at Large, 20/20,* and CNN, and currently hosts the weekly *It's All About Food* show on the Progressive Radio Network. Prior to her work in plant-based nutrition, health, and wellness, Caryn worked as an engineer in the semiconductor industry for twenty years. Caryn is a classically trained singer and performs in opera and musicals in the United States and abroad. She has won two international voice competitions (in France and South Africa). Caryn lives with her partner Gary De Mattei, who is the co-founder of REAL. Together they created *Hartglass & De Mattei, The Swingin' Gourmets,* the first vegan cabaret musical.

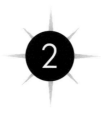

Adele Bloch-Bauer and I

Caryn Hartglass

It was just three days before a long-awaited trip to India and I was feeling lousy. I collapsed on the couch and turned on the TV. This was not typical for me. I don't watch much television. I just needed to lie down, I was so fatigued. On PBS, Charlie Rose was interviewing Ron Lauder. They were talking about the *Adele Bloch-Bauer I*, Gustav Klimt's painting that Lauder had just purchased for a record $135,000,000. It was on display at the Neue, his gallery in Manhattan. I love the work of Gustav Klimt. Although at the time it was not one of my preferred pieces, I felt an immediate obsession to see it. For some reason I thought this would be my only chance to see the "Woman in Gold." Since I was flying to India in a few days I didn't have much time.

The afternoon before leaving for the airport, I took the subway to the gallery. I had about fifteen minutes to spend inside. I stood in front of the *Adele Bloch-Bauer* painting and it brought me to profound tears. I could not explain it. The painting was incredibly beautiful, very large, impressive, and sparkling with lots of gold leaf. But that did not justify my tears. I could not understand what I was feeling. I looked around at the four other Klimt paintings in the room. They were all so lovely. Klimt's *Birch Forest* had me entranced. But when I returned my gaze to the *Adele Bloch-Bauer*, I felt an energy that pierced my soul. All I could do was cry. It was embarrassing. The room was crowded with people. I was out of time and quickly left the building. I had a flight to catch.

That night I flew to India on Aeroflot Airlines. It was a long, unpleasant flight. The flight attendants were grumpy. Still, I was excited about getting to India and it was hard to fall asleep so I tried to watch the movies on board. One of them was *Ocean's Twelve*. I had seen it before and was barely watching it. Toward the end I looked up and saw the actor Andy Garcia sitting at his desk in the casino. I recognized the bottom portion of the painting hanging behind him.

It was the same painting I was standing in front of just hours before, bawling my eyes out, the *Adele Bloch-Bauer*. I did not notice the painting the first time I saw the film. But now I could not help but recognize it. Why was I drawn to this painting? I was spooked.

My condition grew worse while in India. My belly was getting larger and more uncomfortable. The fatigue persisted and my legs were swelling. The problem had begun about a year before. I thought the fibroids I was told I had for many years were getting larger. I went to a new gynecologist in August who wanted me to have a hysterectomy. I had been resisting having surgery but now I was ready. I did not want to wait any longer.

As soon as I got home I scheduled surgery for a few days later. I required a blood transfusion first because of the anemia. After the operation, when I was recovering in my hospital room, my surgeon came to speak with me.

I will never forget that moment. He stood in front of my hospital bed. He spoke quickly and with a serious tone, telling me I had ovarian cancer. He had performed a total hysterectomy and an appendectomy. I was still getting off the anesthesia but his words were clear. He believed he had gotten it all. He said I would need chemotherapy and with this treatment about 90 percent of patients are cured.

CANCER? Me? What? How could I have cancer? I had been pursuing a healthy lifestyle most of my life. At fifteen, I decided I didn't want to kill animals and stopped eating meat and chicken. I eliminated fish a few years later and when I was thirty years old I became a vegan, giving up dairy and eggs. When I discovered that humans did not have to eat nonhuman animals to live, I began reading about and understanding the effects our food choices have not only on nonhuman animals, but also on health and the environment. I wanted to share what I was learning with everyone around me. Healthy plant food was my life! I ran the nonprofit EarthSave International as Executive Director for over eight years. During that time I produced the Taste of Health Food Festival, an all-vegan event with lectures, food demos, and exhibits at Lincoln Center in Manhattan, for five years in a row, with five to ten thousand attendees each year. I hosted lectures featuring the experts in health and plant-based nutrition, read their books, and kept up with research.

I was a healthy vegan. I thought I was invincible. For most of my life, until my belly started growing, I had tons of energy and always felt great. I rarely came down with a cold. After thinking hard, I realized my problem had begun when I was a teenager, but I did not acknowledge it until now. When I began menstruating my periods were always very heavy. This led me to use lots of tampons, often three supers at a time since I was in high school. Tampons contain dioxin and I was getting a big dose, which must have aggravated the problem I had even more. Add to that all the dairy I was consuming as a vegetarian until I went vegan. Dairy consumption is linked to breast, prostate, and ovarian cancers. I believe I was living with a problem for a long time and it was manageable because I had a great diet and a positive attitude toward life. But by the time I was forty-eight years old, something had gone out of balance and the cancer had grown.

During my recovery in the hospital my surgeon would call me by phone in addition to coming to the hospital to check on me. He could not help but notice during the surgery how clean I was inside, with very little fat. Afterwards, he kept asking me for advice on diet and nutrition! So, from my hospital bed, I lectured him and the nurses who were interested about healthy eating. Somehow I knew I would be all right.

Once at home, I began researching information about ovarian cancer. I contacted some of the medical doctors I was close to in the plant-based food movement. While speaking with my friend John Robbins, founder of EarthSave, the organization I worked for, and author of the best seller, *Diet for a New America*, he asked me if I had been dreaming. I told him I hadn't been because I had not been sleeping well for a long time. Then, several nights later, I had a dream with John in it. There were lots of aspects to the dream but the important part for this story is that I saw a very tall, slim woman holding my one-year-old niece. She was so tall we couldn't see the baby.

Three days after the dream, I went to Memorial Sloan-Kettering for a consultation with one of their top gynecologic oncologists. I was sitting in the waiting room with my mother and saw a woman who looked like the tall person in my dream! I got up to take a closer look. She had a purse with the *Adele Bloch-Bauer* pattern on it! It blew my mind. What was my connection to this painting?

John Robbins led me to the Block Center in Evanston, Illinois for chemotherapy. It was a wonderful place and almost made having chemotherapy pleasurable. I called it the Club Med of chemotherapy. I also felt lucky to have so many wonderful people on my side. My friend, colleague, and nutrition expert Dr. Joel Fuhrman recommended that I consume two green juices, two salads (one blended) and have something steamed for dinner like Brussels sprouts. So began my project to cram cruciferous veggies. The Block Center recommended a long list of nutraceuticals to take during treatment. Some were to prevent nausea; some were for fighting cancer and to support my immune system. I committed to taking the supplements, and I had a green juice every day, made with dark leafy-green vegetables combined with other plant foods like celery, cucumber, lemon, and ginger. I avoided sugar, white-flour foods, and sugary fruits. I stuck with berries. My intention was to beat the cancer and to do that I had to supercharge my immune system.

There was a small residual mass remaining after my surgery that was found on my PET scan before I started chemotherapy, giving me an ovarian cancer staging of IIIC. Everyone told me the chemo would take care of it. Unfortunately, it had grown during the treatment and now I needed to have another surgery to remove it.

The doctor who did the first surgery performed the second in March 2007 but he couldn't find anything. He said it was possible to have a false positive from a PET scan. I wanted to believe I was cancer-free but for the next three months I did not feel well. After another scan in June 2007, the mass was still there and had doubled in size.

It was time to find the right surgeon that I felt I could trust with my life. A very close friend recommended Dr. Joel Bauer because she had known someone who had had cancer in a similar location and liked him very much. When I met with him I knew he was the one for the job. I had met with other surgeons who did not think I could be cured and that they could only buy me time. Dr. Bauer was confident that he and his team could make me well. He was the doctor I was looking for.

I had my third surgery at Mt. Sinai on Friday, July 13, 2007, and it was a success. The surgery lasted about two hours and the tumor mass was removed. My sister Lori had flown in from Florida to be with me and she stayed at my parents' home on Long Island. She woke up with a start on Sunday morning, July 15, at about 5:00 a.m. All at once, the meaning behind my dreams and emotions surrounding Gustav Klimt's painting, the *Adele Bloch-Bauer* had dawned on her. She got up and turned on the computer just to verify that the name of the painting was indeed "Bloch-Bauer." She felt like she was going to burst. She had to tell someone, but it was too early. She waited a couple of hours and then called me. As she shared her experience, she reminded me who the two doctors were who played a big role in saving my life, Dr. Block at the Block Center and Dr. Bauer, my surgeon, at Mt. Sinai. Block and Bauer, Block-Bauer — and then I got it — BLOCH-BAUER. The painting was telling me the doctors I needed to use to save my life. It confirmed that I had made the right choice.

I returned to the Block Center for more chemotherapy from September 2007 until the end of December 2007. I was given an aggressive treatment with the intent to cure me. My doctors were amazed at how well I was managing. I did have symptoms, such as fatigue, slight nausea from time to time, and lightheadedness when my red blood cells were dropping. But overall, I did very well — "sailed through it" were the words of one of my doctors. All through the surgeries and chemotherapy I continued working, running EarthSave, and living my life, which included performing.

Finally done with treatments, I celebrated with a trip. I flew to Florida in January 2008 to visit with family and then continued on to Costa Rica. On the flight from Fort Lauderdale to Costa Rica I was intently reading a book. All of a sudden, I wondered what film might be playing and chuckled to myself that it might be *Ocean's Twelve*. I knew it couldn't be because the movie was too old. I looked up and it was *Ocean's Thirteen*! Just a few seconds later, I saw the scene with Andy Garcia in his office at the casino. Only this time there was another Klimt painting there, the *Fritza Riedler*. I remembered my life partner, Gary De Mattei, telling me that the patterns of the Egyptian eyes in the dress of the *Adele Bloch-Bauer* resembled the patterns and colors of the tumor on my PET scan. Fritza Riedler was wearing a pure white dress in her portrait, symbolic for me of being cancer-free and well again.

KATHY STOKES, president of KSM Communications LLC, is a business communications consultant. She helps her clients get their messages heard, whether their audiences are consumers, businesses, employee groups, or policymakers. Kathy serves a wide variety of clients on a range of communications projects. Clients have included Ernst & Young, AARP, the Women's Institute for a Secure Retirement, the Employee Benefit Research Institute, Altarum Institute, MetLife Mature Market Institute, Heinz Family Philanthropies, and Walt Disney World. Kathy has written numerous publications on a range of financial planning topics. She is the author of a high school textbook, *Insurance Operations*, published in 2013.

Prior to launching her own firm in 2006, Kathy was on the founding team of the Brookings Institution's Retirement Security Project. Other companies she has worked for include the Employee Benefit Research Institute, the American Savings Education Council, and Ernst & Young.

Kathy holds a bachelor's degree in Rhetoric and Communication from the University of Pittsburgh and a master's degree in American Government from Johns Hopkins University. Her master's thesis was on pensions and retirement security.

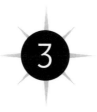

3

Silver Linings

Kathy Stokes

Cancer sucks.

When I told my fourteen-year-old daughter, Cailyn, that I was writing this essay and didn't know how to start it, she simply advised, "Why not start out by saying how much cancer sucks?" And she was right. There's no shrinking away from this cold fact. It's terrifying, debilitating, and will likely put your body through more than it's ever had to endure.

If you're reading this because you've been diagnosed, let me say right up front that I'm so sorry. That really sucks. If you're like me, you'll appreciate hearing that.

But it doesn't all suck. (Cailyn went on to advise me to include this part, too.) I found in my seventeen-month battle with breast cancer many silver linings. For example, I renewed a loving and supportive

45

relationship with my three sisters that years and family turmoil had withered away. I had more than one hundred people who called themselves My Army who helped in myriad ways, from carting my kids around to feeding us, accompanying me to chemo appointments, walking the dogs, and just checking in to let me know I wasn't forgotten.

I found a way to get through, and picked up some useful insights along the way. Here are five of them; pick one or all. Any of them will make the road a little less rocky.

Insight #1: People won't know what to say — give them that.

I'll bet you fifty dollars right now that most of the people you tell will respond by telling you about someone else who has breast cancer. This is not helpful! You don't want to feel like just another number when this monumental rock gets dropped on you. Looking back, I wish I had the nerve to tell people that their stories weren't helpful. But I just let them keep coming at me, and at times I just wanted to crawl under my covers. I even had people tell me that at least I had a "good" cancer! Trust me when I tell you there's no such thing as a good cancer. Understand that your news is a big blow to whomever you tell. They won't know what to say for the most part. My dear friend Michelle was the most forthright about it. She hugged me and then admitted that she didn't know what to say. I suggested she say, "I'm sorry; that really sucks. What can I do to help?" That's exactly what she said, and it felt loving and supportive.

***Insight* #2: You'll have more than one doctor.**

You will deal with three or more doctors, depending on your specific diagnosis. I had my breast surgeon, whom I had been seeing for fifteen years because of my particularly dense breast tissue that called for special attention. This is the doctor who diagnosed me and performed a bilateral (double) mastectomy. Then, I had to find an oncologist for post-surgical treatment and a plastic surgeon for breast reconstruction.

I was fortunate that my breast surgeon's office had a nurse navigator. Find out if one exists in your doctor's office. My nurse navigator Lorna was a godsend (and another silver lining). Not only did she help me find an oncologist and a plastic surgeon, but she advocated for getting my surgery done quickly, helped me understand what to expect, and became a trusted resource and friend.

Meet with your doctors and get a feel for how they'll handle your case. Some oncology offices have big rooms where multiple chemo patients get treatment at the same time. Others have private rooms. There are pros and cons to both. I went with the private room, which was great when I had a friend there with me. It felt pretty lonely when I was on my own, though, and I sort of wished there was another patient sitting next to me. Not even to talk, necessarily. Just to know I wasn't in it alone.

Insight #3: **Accept help willingly.**

I am fiercely independent (bull-headed could be a little closer to the truth). I've always chafed at having to ask for help. But that went out the door fast once I received my diagnosis.

At the time, I was a forty-six-year-old, self-employed single mom to eleven-year-old twins. When my doctor sat me down and told me I had breast cancer, my very first thought was, "How am I going to do this on my own?" And at the time, I didn't have any idea what my treatment had in store for me.

My dearest friend Kim picked up the mantle without hesitation. She created an online support portal through which friends could sign up to help with specific needs. And they came out in droves! (Another silver lining.) We put a cooler on my porch for people to drop off meals several times a week. I left the dog leashes outside so people could come by, call the dogs out through the dog door, and get them their exercise. My kids got rides to their activities. I got rides to my appointments. And my ex readily took the kids when chemo treatments left me with no energy.

The bottom line is you can't go it alone. Don't try to be a hero by continuing to manage life the way you did before your diagnosis; you're already a hero for the journey you're on.

Insight #4: Chemo? Ice, socks, and a razor are your friends.

I endured twenty weeks of chemo and another year of antibody infusions. You already know that cancer sucks. Chemo, at least for me, was the worst part of it all. I reacted badly to my first treatment so the nurses slowed down future infusions. That meant seven- to eight-hour treatments, hooked up through a port implanted in my chest. I would feel okay the first day or two following treatment, but then I'd get nauseated and dizzy, and not start feeling better until a new chemo round was due. It was a trying and rather vicious cycle. I never vomited, but I almost always felt like I would. I lost twenty pounds through the ordeal.

One of the side effects of chemo is painful mouth lesions. I found I could avoid or at least reduce them by keeping my mouth cold during chemo. I constantly had ice in my mouth (I tried popsicles but they just made me feel sick to my stomach). The cold creates a barrier so the chemo can't be absorbed in your mouth. Trust me on this one; chewing ice beats sore gums and cheeks by miles.

Another side effect is cold feet. Find yourself some warm socks or slippers to wear during your chemo infusions. You'll thank me later.

My hair started falling out about three weeks into my treatment. It was an emotionally painful experience to grab a handful of my thick hair and have it fall into my lap. It was physically painful, too. My scalp really hurt where the hair was coming from. My girlfriend Laura took me to my hairdresser, and he graciously shaved my head. I went to pay him and he told me to hold my money until he could give me a new hairstyle. (More silver linings.) I wore a cotton cap to bed to help protect my head from the discomfort of lying on pillows. It worked well.

Insight #5: Understand the implant process.

As a relatively young and single woman, I didn't hesitate in my decision to undergo breast reconstruction following my bilateral mastectomy. If you go this route, and I'd recommend it from my experience, there are a few things to understand.

First, your mastectomy and initial reconstruction will happen in the same surgery. The plastic surgeon will implant placeholders that will stretch your skin to allow for the implants. Mine felt like turtle shells under my skin. They are uncomfortable but you get used to them. Once you're healed from surgery, you'll visit the plastic surgeon periodically to "fill" the placeholders and stretch the skin. It's not painful per se, but you'll feel uncomfortable for a few days after.

You'll have a choice between using your own fat and going with implants. I chose the latter because it was far less invasive. I assumed that I'd have scars but at least I'd have even breasts. After healing, it turned out that I wasn't even and I could see the ripples of the implants under my skin. I'm kind of stuck with the ripples, but not with the lopsidedness. I had another surgery to remove excess skin to even them out. I'm pleased with the results. Oh, and if you find yourself without nipples like I did, Google a guy named Vinnie in Baltimore. He does magnificent, 3D nipple and areola tattoos.

For me, the biggest silver lining of being diagnosed with an aggressive form of breast cancer, going through three surgeries, losing my hair (all of it, ladies) and at times my will, and enduring the horrible side effects of chemo was watching how my children, Cailyn and Aidan, handled it all. They were a tremendous support for me, all the while keeping up with their schoolwork and their activities. Every single day, and every day since, Aïdan asks, "How are you feeling, Mom?" I know these aren't just words. He is growing up to be an empathetic, caring young man. They both weathered the storm and are stronger for it. I am, too.

Trust that you will find silver linings amid the dark clouds. And you may find a will to try something new or something you've always wanted to do. I've since joined one band as a singer and started a second one, and even got to record an original song. Plus, I had the opportunity to meet Vice President Biden and share my story with over seven hundred health-care advocates. And I've learned that life's too short to get caught up in fear and regret. Discovering that in itself is worth the pain and suffering.

Yes, cancer sucks. But it isn't all dark clouds. Find your silver linings, and appreciate every one of them. I hope the insights I've shared tell you something new and useful. If so, consider it a silver lining.

RACHAEL YAHNE is a writer, blogger, cancer survivor and the author of HerAfter.com, a women's site about beautiful, conscious living. After years as a fashion journalist, Rachael now writes lifestyle articles on happiness, love, beauty, finding purpose and living a fulfilling life not just after cancer, but through all of life's big struggles. Her work has been featured on Huffington Post, Yahoo!, The Seattle Times, BlogHer, and a variety of online magazines. For more information, visit her Web site, HerAfter.com.

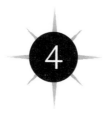

Forgiveness on the Other Side of the World

Rachael Yahne

I walk into the hotel room, its crisp sheets folded so strictly, its tile floors slapping back on my sandals, and I drop my bags in the center of the room. It's been ten hours of weary travel and ten years of wait and worry to get to this place. I open the patio door to a half-moon private balcony that sits on a cliff, overlooking the cove beach of this tiny Greek isle. Out ahead, there is only miles of sand held delicately by endless blue sea. The sun hits my face, I smell the ocean below, and I break into tears. *What unadulterated, uninhibited bliss*, I think. *I made it.* On my knees in the sea-salt afternoon air, I weep and I weep and I weep.

It's been ten years, and I'm still finding ways to forgive you, cancer.

I was diagnosed at seventeen. At the time, it was easy not to harbor any anger at the very thing trying to kill me. I had questions, sure, but no anger. It felt like fighting a ghost I couldn't see, like it was sucking my existence out from within, but I still had a firm enough grip to hold on. It was even easy to sacrifice certain aspects of life — school, hair, being a teenager — in order to know that someday I'd be back to living again, without cancer, without restrictions. I could manage to forgive cancer for things like making my mom and I live apart from my brothers and dad while I did treatment, since there was nothing in our hometown capable of saving me. Our hometown hospitals had not the treatments nor the doctors to cure such an advanced stage of sickness.

But after the chemo was over, I found new angers, new problems that weren't so easy to forgive. What no one ever tells you about fighting cancer is that the fight never really ends. You can kill it, but for the rest of your life you've either got the fears or the sacrifices, or at the very least the yearly check-ups with your doctor to remind you that yes, it happened. It's still happening. How ironic that the one to stick by your side every day of your life is the ghost that tried to kill you. No matter how hard you fought, it will find new ways to break you down, and you have to keep fighting.

This truth became all the more evident in college, years after chemo, when I started having my first serious relationships. After a month or so of dating someone new, I'd feel the need to come clean and tell him I'd had cancer as a teen. But that required telling him the potential dangers involved in spending his life with me, because it could come back, or keep me from having kids, or have other effects on us. The first person I told seemed inspired rather than distraught, and the exchange gave me a bit of hubris. Later potential partners weren't so confident. It was a deal breaker for them; they'd say they couldn't handle it or they'd be unwilling to look at pictures of me bald. I can't be mad at them, sometimes cancer is bigger than some people can handle. But could I be mad at cancer then? How can I forgive cancer for making me have *that* conversation? The only way I could forgive cancer is by being grateful it got the wrong people out of the way.

There was also the white medical mask I had to wear to college in the winter. With my immune system still quite low, it was easier (and safer) to simply wear a mask to classes during flu season, especially if someone in class was sick. Surprisingly, it's much easier to get past flu season relatively unscathed than to get past all the strange looks, all the fear in the eyes of the passersby, as if *I* was the problem.

Over the years it's left scars and marks and taken away freedom and even sometimes joy. It's taken my family from me many, many times. In so many ways it's taken my naïveté too, and with so many goodbyes to people and parts of myself, forgiveness isn't always right there like an old friend to help me through. In my early twenties, I went so far as to push my health to its edge and endanger my own physical and mental safety, all in a vain attempt to be normal, reckless like everyone else. It didn't work and I hated myself for what I *wanted* to blame cancer for making me do. Forgiveness of myself turned out to be the hardest of all.

Forgiveness. It's so vital to our well-being, and yet it's so difficult to grasp. What do I have to give up of myself to move on? As if I haven't given cancer enough already. What do I have to hand over to make it work: My ego? My expectations? My own wants and desires? Fairness? It's not so cut-and-dried like we were taught in childhood. That which is lost in the transaction isn't always just a few crumbs of cookie. Maybe I'd been attempting to demand fairness in exchange for my forgiveness, but cancer simply doesn't work that way.

Then again, sometimes just when I start to feel that cancer is all ugliness and greed and all it does is take, take, take, I'll find myself in conversation with another survivor about the beauty of simply sitting in silence, experiencing the flow of time. Or how blessed we are to have eyebrows again — EYEBROWS! So blessed we'd never criticize or berate them. There are emotions and conversations I find easier to have with others who've faced cancer, profound conversations that are so enlightening, I can only think of them as acts of worship to life itself.

And there are other gifts cancer gives me. I believe now that I've got a love deeper and more connected than most people, *because* of the conversation that cancer forced upon us. We became closer through experiencing it. When someone commits to raising your kids without you should cancer come back and you can't fight it, love explodes like fireworks big and bright and miraculous before you. It takes a really big love to choose someone else over fear or fairness.

I like best the gifts cancer gives me in and of myself, too. I like the scars on my arms and my waist, I like to spend time with my body and to study it and to think about all it's done for me. I like to take special care of it, inside and out, treasure it as if it's like a temple. I can only laugh when my closest friends panic about voluntarily cutting off two inches of their hair. I like the signs of my own aging, because I know I'm lucky to be having them. The wrinkles and freckles, like little kisses from the wisdom of this planet. I even like the fear, at least sometimes, because it deepens my awareness of *this* moment, a moment when there is nothing to fear just yet, a moment when I'm still alive and cancer is still not. These are the kinds of moments that make it easy to love cancer, as ugly and greedy as it is.

Especially, perhaps, this day, on the balcony in Greece. It's the celebratory trip to commemorate a decade of survivorship and all that I'd been through with cancer, because of cancer, for cancer. My partner and I are at the beginning of our ten-day trip for a ten-year anniversary after ten hours of travel — yes, tens everywhere in the magical way the universe loves to joke with us — and it's our first day in Greece at this beautiful hotel. On the agenda: absolutely nothing. Nothing but stillness, sunshine, praying to the ocean by soaking in it, praising the sun for letting me greet it again when it might have set forever on me so long ago. It's about feeling the sand on our toes, the time in our bodies, the gratitude for having made it here. Nothing but existing in one of the most beautiful places on the planet and here I am, filled with bliss.

In fact, bliss is shining out so brightly from my heart, it meets the sunlight and blinds everything around me. Bliss so strong and so sweet, it makes the sound of my crying like a rich symphony. I'm surrounded by it, in a safe little bubble of timelessness, and no words of gratitude or appreciation or joy could ever describe it, so I just feel it in every inch of my scarred body, of my broken and healed heart, through every corner and within every vein. It's just enrapturing bliss so much so it becomes all of me, and I am only light and love. And in being light and love, and letting the bliss become so big it encompasses me, I can only forgive again and again. Gratitude makes room for nothing but light. Oh what bright bliss! I whisper an airy "thank you" out loud to the universe. I'm so lucky, I'm so, so lucky to be here.

Forgiveness isn't always on the other side of the world, though. I see now it's not something you run toward, it's something you look inwardly to find. Forgiveness is waiting just inside our hearts, but our own fears and wants keep us from reaching out for its hand and climbing to the other side. But when we stop keeping track of what's fair and what's not, and stop asking life to give as much as we give, we can take a look around at all we really have. Forgiveness isn't about saying "this transaction isn't even, but I'll move past it anyway." It's realizing that life *only* gives and gives and gives in experience and lessons, and those lessons will open you up to feel more bliss than you ever thought possible. Such bliss it brings you to your knees in tears.

Forgiveness is the humble realization that you will never have as much to give to life as it does to you, and that all you can do is simply be grateful to have ever gotten at all.

And so my cancer, my forgiveness and I go forward into gratitude. We are lucky to be here. We are so, so lucky to have each other.

LIZ LANGE pioneered "maternity chic" by creating stylish, body conscious clothing for pregnant women. After working at *Vogue Magazine*, Liz developed the idea for a sophisticated and slim-fitting collection of maternity clothing. In 1997, out of a one-room office, she created Liz Lange Maternity, changing forever the face of maternity fashions. She has dressed every major pregnant celebrity, forging licensing deals with Nike and Target.

Liz Lange Maternity for Target is the exclusive maternity department at all Target locations and offers affordable maternity pieces, from flattering jeans and T-shirts to on-trend dresses and swimsuits. In 2012, Liz celebrated her tenth anniversary of Liz Lange Maternity for Target, marking a decade of helping expecting moms dress stylishly on a budget. Liz is also author of *Liz Lange's Maternity Style: How to Look Fabulous During the Most Fashion-Challenged Time*.

As a retail and fashion pioneer Liz also developed a ready-to-wear collection for HSN, Completely Me ™ by Liz Lange. Liz is the only maternity designer to be a member of the prestigious Council of Fashion Designers of America and is a regular contributor and fashion expert to several leading publications and broadcast outlets.

Liz is actively involved in many charities and is a spokesperson for cervical cancer awareness. Most recently she has partnered with Jhpiego, a global health nonprofit dedicated to improving the health of women and families in developing countries, to raise awareness of maternal and child health issues.

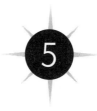

How I Beat Cancer — *My* Way

Liz Lange

(This essay is adapted and updated from a Glamour *magazine article by Liz Lange as told to Shaun Dreisbach and is reprinted with permission.)*

Many cancer survivors say to focus on wellness, make your life Zen, and tell everyone you know so they can help you through it. I am not judging that advice, as I am sure for many it is extremely helpful. But for me personally I wanted to keep it very private. Not because I was ashamed but because I wanted to keep it highly compartmentalized so that other than when I was receiving treatment and speaking to doctors, I could have completely non-cancer experiences and conversations.

So for six years, until I was forty-one years old, I chose to basically tell no one that I had been diagnosed with cervical cancer at age thirty-five. Keeping it a secret might sound crazy to you. After all, people blog about their experiences with cancer, join support groups — every week, it seems, a celebrity comes forward with her incredible cancer story, sharing the details as she lives through it. I know many women find great solace in airing their fears and feeling like they have a huge base of sympathy and support. But for me, *not* talking about my cancer turned out to be what saved me. So this is how I took things — one step at a time.

Step 1: Don't Put Off That Pap

It was the summer of 2001 and things could not have been crazier. I had a new baby — eight-month-old Alice — and a two-and-a-half-year-old son, Gus, and my four-year-old business designing clothes for pregnant women was taking off in a big way. I had earned a spot at New York's Fashion Week in the fall (which would make me the first-ever maternity designer to show there) and was in the midst of putting together my collection. I was also debuting a brand-new line of pregnancy workout clothes for Nike.

So the last thing I had time for was a trip to the gynecologist. But I was due for a checkup, and for some reason I decided I shouldn't put it off. A week after the test, I got a call from my doctor: "The results of your Pap smear were funny," he said. A follow-up biopsy found that I had dysplasia — abnormal tissue that, left untreated, can be a precursor to cervical cancer. A simple procedure removed it, and I was assured it wasn't a huge deal. I was literally breezing out the door after the procedure when my doctor called out after me, "It's standard practice to test the actual dysplasia. We'll have the results in about a week." To me, the problem had already been taken care of.

Step 2: Imagine the Worst

I was in the car with my mother more than a week later, coming back from a wedding in East Hampton, when my cell phone buzzed with a message from my doctor. I checked my voice mail at work; he had tried to reach me there, too.

And that's when I knew I had cancer. It was Columbus Day — why try to reach me twice on a holiday if there was no news to tell?

My face flushed and I felt as if I was going to throw up. I dialed the doctor and he immediately came to the phone. "Well, I don't have good news . . ." he began. I couldn't hear anymore. "I'm sorry, I can't talk about this!" I said, and handed the phone to my mother even though she was at the wheel. He didn't want to discuss something so upsetting while she was driving, so he quickly relayed just two things: I had cervical cancer, and he'd made an appointment for me with a gynecologic oncologist first thing the next morning.

For two hours I imagined myself getting sick, losing my hair, and dying. Cancer has always been my worst fear. Even as a child I was terrified of it. I remember getting marker on my hand once and running to my mom, panicked, saying I'd found a spot; I must have heard something about skin cancer. At one point, my parents had to ask my pediatrician to explain to me how rare cancer is in kids.

My mother and I were nearly silent for the rest of the drive, except every few minutes she would say, in a stunned, far-off way, "We are going to get all the best doctors."

That night I couldn't bear walking into my apartment and having to face my husband and, especially, my kids. I was overwhelmed, and the thought of seeing them — and knowing that their lives hinged on the outcome — was more than I could emotionally handle. So instead I went to my mother's house. We called the doctor again and got more details, which were somewhat reassuring: My cancer was treatable. Only then did I call my husband; I sobbed hysterically as I told him the news.

Step 3: Find a Kind Doctor

Another silent car ride. This time it was with my husband, who was coming with me to meet the oncologist. When the doctor walked in to see us, I blurted out, "Am I going to die?"

"*Die*? Of course you're not going to die!" he said. He recommended a radical hysterectomy to remove the cancer on my cervix and any abnormal cells that may have spread, but he also encouraged me to get more opinions. What a nightmare that was. One doctor assaulted me with survival statistics and then had his staff give us literature on the hospital's chapel services. Another, who was supposed to be brilliant, treated me like Cancer Patient Number 607. I felt so vulnerable that any insensitivity seemed like cruelty. After two weeks of doctor shopping, I went back to my original oncologist. He had great credentials, but most of all, he had heart.

His optimism helped whenever I found myself having melodramatic but very real thoughts. I'd look at my kids and think, *They're so innocent; they don't know.* I'd wander into their rooms in the middle of the night to be close to them, and I'd just stand there thinking, *They* need *me.*

Step 4: Keep the News a Secret

By the time I scheduled the surgery, I had told my sister, my husband, my parents, two friends, and my cousin about my illness. Before the operation I also told two key business associates, who would have to handle things for me while I recovered. But most people in my life — other friends, my employees — had no idea. Why did I decide to keep quiet? The most honest answer I can give is that it was simply too painful for me to talk about. Every time I tried, my face would turn bright red, I'd break down in tears, and I wouldn't be able to get the word *cancer* out of my mouth.

It was hard for me even to admit to *myself* that I had cancer. I made sure I did everything I could to get better physically, yet emotionally I was practically not dealing with it. Some of that was denial, I'm sure, but mainly it helped me function. If a lot of people had known about my condition, I constantly would have been peppered with questions about how the treatment was going, or how I was holding up — and that would have just mired me in the problem when I wanted to concentrate on beating my cancer.

I also worried about what the news could do to my company. I thought, *I'm supposed to be the queen of maternity chic, and here I am about to have a hysterectomy!* I feared it would be bad for the brand that I had worked so hard to create. I like being seen as a strong, successful woman. I couldn't bear people thinking of me as anything but that.

Step 5: Have Chemo While Landing a Huge Business Deal

It took two weeks to recover from the hysterectomy, but it appeared that the cancer had not spread. Still, my oncologist recommended a five-week course of chemotherapy, and my radiologist advised eight weeks of radiation. It was aggressive, but it would dramatically reduce the risk of recurrence. I was ready to do whatever it took. Thankfully, the chemo wouldn't cause my hair to fall out. Outwardly, at least, I would be the same old Liz.

Not having my employees know about my diagnosis and treatment helped keep life normal, which was a huge comfort to me. I could go into the office and not worry that they weren't telling me things or not giving me work because they didn't want to stress me out. In fact, I went for radiation treatment at the hospital every morning before work, and no one in the office found out. Hiding it did get stressful sometimes. Once I bumped into a friend of my mother's in the hospital lobby. "Oh, Liz, what are you doing here?" she asked. I stumbled and made up a lie about visiting a friend who had just had a baby. But I was panicked that I almost had been exposed.

Once a week I also had chemotherapy; I'd have an IV put in my arm and then sit for two to three hours while the medicine dripped into me. My sister came with me every time. We'd sit and chat and she'd bring fashion magazines for us to flip through. But we never, ever discussed cancer.

In the middle of my treatment, I had a launch party to

present my Liz Lange for Nike maternity activewear line to a select group of New York editors. It was a huge moment in my career, but I was exhausted and weak from having chemo and radiation that morning. I remember sitting on the floor of my shower, too tired to stand, and being unable to lift my arms to shampoo my hair. I have no idea how, but I managed to do my hair, put on my makeup, and get through the event. To cover the fact that I wasn't as energetic as usual, I told colleagues that I was getting over the flu. But no one could tell how sick I really was.

A few weeks later I got a call from Target. They wanted me to fly to Minneapolis to discuss launching a new maternity line. I was beyond excited, but I couldn't take a day off from radiation, so I invented an excuse to put them off until I had a weeklong break in my treatment. When I finally negotiated the deal, I thought, *I never knew I had it in me to do something like this — let alone with cancer.*

Step 6: Finally Tell the World

When I reached the six-year mark of being cancer-free, I finally began to feel like it was close to being behind me. It seemed like the right time to go public. A million times over the prior six years I was asked, "When are you going to have another baby? You're the poster child for your brand." I'd say, "I don't have time — my business is my third child." But that wasn't the whole truth. I began to realize that being completely open could help people — and that was the most important thing. I'm inspired every day by strong women who are talking about cancer, like Katie Couric, who lost her husband to colon cancer. I knew that if I could raise awareness about cervical cancer, I should.

In all my years of going to the ob-gyn, it had never occurred to me how crucial regular Pap smears were (I think today they have an even better test than the Pap). I have to confess that before my diagnosis, I wasn't even sure what the test screened for — ovarian or cervical cancer. I don't want you, or any other woman who reads this story, to put important screening tests off. The Pap literally saved my life. And I knew I'd feel guilty if I didn't do all I could to save someone else's.

I was very close to the Editor-in-Chief of *Glamour* magazine, Cindi Leive, and I decided to tell my story to her readers first. But that really opened the floodgates. I also told my story to *People* magazine. I then became a spokesperson for National Cervical Cancer Awareness Month and did a media tour, where I told my story to as many media outlets as possible in the hopes of making sure that all women saw their health-care providers regularly.

Today it's been fifteen years since that awful Columbus Day diagnosis. To be honest, I even sometimes forget that I am a "cancer survivor." I'm just me.

BARBARA MUSSER is a respected and inspiring intimacy and sexuality speaker, educator, coach, facilitator, and author. She was diagnosed with breast cancer in 1989 as a young single woman. She married and had a child after treatment. Since then, she has worked with thousands of women, couples, and healthcare professionals, specializing in creating programs to help heal the trauma of cancer treatments to femininity, intimacy, sexuality, and relationships. She is the founder and CEO of Sexy After Cancer. She is the author of Sexy After Cancer: Meeting Your Inner Aphrodite on the Breast Cancer Journey. She is a member of AASECT, the American Association of Sex Educators, Counselors and Therapists, and ISSWSH, the International Society for the Study of Women's Sexual Health.

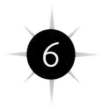

6

The Long and Winding Road: Waking Up to Beauty and Sexiness

Barbara Musser

On my thirty-seventh birthday I heard the words, "You have breast cancer." Everything changed in that moment as I came face to face with my mortality. I was newly single, dating, had just received a promotion and a raise at work, and had moved into a sweet new home. Suddenly, none of that mattered. I had no context for this and no way to navigate all the changes and decisions.

Ironically, my mother and sister arrived the next day to visit. We wanted to explore the northern California coast, laugh, and have fun. I was hoping to heal an emotional rift between Mom and me, and I really needed her to hold me and comfort me. She couldn't talk about my cancer; instead, she simply said that she knew I'd be fine. The rift healed that week when I realized that she was doing her best and that I needed to find other emotional and spiritual support. Once I did that, I was able to receive the love that she offered. I began to learn that healing and love often come in unexpected ways.

Many aspects of my life shifted during treatment. New friends appeared to listen, hold my hand, and cry with me. I created a healing team for the journey and spent a lot of time meditating, doing yoga, and praying. I left my big corporate job to devote myself to activities that fed my soul and made the world a better place. My journey turned inward as I dug deep for resources that I hoped I had, to heal and make meaning of my life. I was in completely new territory and had no map, and I trusted that this was how it was meant to be.

Initially I thought that my romantic life was over. After all, who would want to be with a woman who was clearly "damaged goods"? Our culture emphasizes physical perfection as a measure of a woman's worth and desirability. I wasn't perfect before cancer and now I felt I was much less so by those standards. Though I wasn't willing to throw in the towel, I didn't know how to heal this. And I certainly didn't want to face a life without romance, intimacy, or sex. The idea of devoting myself to a monastic spiritual path crossed my mind briefly as I contemplated the future. That felt extreme and scary.

Then it dawned on me that it was time to look inside to see what I'm made of and what it meant to live my best life. Cancer literally woke me up to *me*, and I took myself on in a way that I never had before. I searched for resources to help heal my heart, my mind, and my spirit. This was a long time ago and there weren't many resources then because people weren't living a long time after their diagnosis. I was determined to live long and well and to discover how.

One thing I knew was that I wasn't ready to give up on love, romance, and sex, and that a life of celibacy wasn't in the cards for me. That meant that I had to heal my self-esteem and body image, to learn how to accept and love myself, changed as I was by cancer and its treatments. Little did I know that this inner inquiry and healing would become the basis for my life's work. I didn't realize that my journey would have value for others on the path, or that I had the courage to heal these deep wounds. I never imagined that twenty-seven years later, I'd be an inspiration for women to heal and grow, to thrive and live and love after cancer came into their lives.

You know that adage about making God laugh by making plans? Gradually I learned to laugh along with God and to recognize that my previously planned life wasn't my best life going forward. The vision that I'd marry, have lots of babies, and live in a happy and tranquil home with a big family, evaporated. The opportunities and adventures that appeared have been extraordinary. It amazes me that they came as a result of my cancer diagnosis. I'm not saying that cancer is a gift because no one wants it. I am saying that I used cancer as a turning point in my life. It wasn't always pleasant or easy.

It wasn't easy to begin to accept and love myself. I read voraciously, attended workshops and psychotherapy and support groups, did yoga, meditated, prayed, and dragged myself through treatment. Sometimes I wonder how I actually managed to turn my life around. Then I remember that I made good choices about treatment and support, I took really good care of me, and I never gave up on my vision of having a life filled with meaning, love, romance, and satisfying intimacy and sex.

There were many turning points. A major one was when I found my way to powerful personal-growth workshops called "Love, Intimacy and Sexuality." The title was both exciting and terrifying. I didn't know when I signed up that the workshops were clothing optional, which meant that participants had the option to be naked in the workshops. I probably wouldn't have gone if I had known. But there I was and I trusted that this was the right place to be. At first I knew there was no way I'd get naked in a room of one hundred men and women, not with my deformed body. There was no pressure to do so, and on the second day I removed my top, thinking that people would leave the room when they saw me. No one even blinked or stared at me.

During the workshop there were several opportunities to stand in front of the group and share personal experiences. I knew I had to do that, that it would be part of accepting myself as I was, radically changed by cancer and treatments. Naked, I stood in front of the group with my knees shaking and barely breathing because I was so scared. I began to talk about having cancer, surgeries, and radiation, and how I was afraid that no man would want to look at me, much less be with me. People were looking at me, smiling, offering support and love — they were accepting me. I mustered up my courage and asked them to raise their hands if they thought I was still attractive. Almost every hand in the room went up. Then I asked the men to be honest and raise their hand if they'd be interested in dating me. Many hands went up. Then a man sitting near me got on his knees and bowed to me. Soon after, almost everyone in the room did the same.

In that moment, I began to cry and let it sink in that I was beautiful and desirable. Those moments changed my life and my healing began to accelerate. I woke up to the beauty of my essence.

Many people approached me during breaks to offer words of love and support. Five women came to share that they also had breast cancer and that I had opened the possibility of healing for them as well. The last day of the workshop, six women with breast cancer joined me in standing naked in front of the group, showing ourselves and receiving love and acknowledgment for our courage, beauty, and grace. It was awesome. There wasn't a dry eye in the house.

This was when I realized that the next step on my path was to become a leader of those workshops, and I traveled the world for fifteen years doing that. There were always people there who'd had cancer, and they often began a new part of their journey of healing and becoming open to more love and intimacy in their lives.

Many years ago I became a sex educator to offer resources and tools for people with cancer. It is now possible to overcome sexual challenges, create and enjoy intimacy and sex, and experience pleasure and satisfaction. I often hear that people now have hope in their romantic relationships. And hope heals and helps build bridges to renewed romance, intimacy, and sexuality.

And for me personally? While I was in treatment I met a man and we became lovers. A few years later we married and had a child. What a miracle! Now I'm single again and dating and I know how beautiful and desirable I am. And my mission is that everyone whose life has been touched by cancer can also know how gorgeous, desirable, and sexy they are. Here's to you and your great life!

ALICE HOFFMAN has published twenty-one novels, three books of short fiction, and eight books for children and young adults. Her books have been published in more than twenty translations and more than one hundred foreign editions. Her novels, many of which have been *New York Times* best sellers, have received mention as notable books of the year by the *New York Times*, *Entertainment Weekly*, the *Los Angeles Times*, *Library Journal*, and *People* magazine. Alice's advance from *Survival Lessons* was donated to the Hoffman Breast Center at Mount Auburn Hospital in Cambridge, Massachusetts.

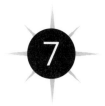

Choose to Accept Sorrow

Alice Hoffman

During my radiation treatment I read *Man's Search for Meaning*. People said, *Isn't that book depressing?* But it wasn't. It was honest. The author, Viktor Frankl, was a psychiatrist who lost nearly everyone he loved in the Holocaust. This fact already makes your problems feel small even if you are in the radiation waiting room. Frankl later developed a theory about tragedy and sorrow, that it is these experiences that make us human and define who we are.

I was looking for an answer in the waiting room. It was the beginning of my search for advice on how to survive. Here is the lesson I learned from Frankl about his time in a concentration camp, an explanation of

how certain people were able to continue on despite
extreme darkness:

*We had to learn ourselves and, furthermore, we had to teach
the despairing men, that it did not really matter what we
expected from life, but rather what life expected from us. We
needed to stop asking about the meaning of life, and instead
to think of ourselves as those who were being questioned by
life — daily and hourly. Our answer must consist, not in talk
and meditation, but in right action and in right conduct. Life
ultimately means taking the responsibility to find the right
answer to its problems and to fulfill the task which it constantly
sets for each individual.*

We are all responsible for our actions, and our
reactions. We are responsible for how we respond
to situations we cannot control. I could not run
away from my circumstances, or control the path of
my disease, but I could control what I did with my
experience of that illness. I chose to become a fund-
raiser for breast cancer. That was the right answer to
my problem. As a matter of fact, I think it may be the
rightest and best answer I've ever found. When you
help others, your own troubles aren't as heavy. In fact,
you can fold them like a handkerchief and place them

in your pocket. They're still there, but they're not the only thing you carry.

A self-described "everyday woman," B A R B A R A D E L I N S K Y was born and raised in Boston, Massachusetts. She received degrees in Psychology and Sociology, married, and had three sons. She wrote a book, and it sold. So she wrote another, and another. In 1994, the year both her ninth and tenth novels were published, Barbara was also diagnosed with breast cancer. Like any "everyday woman," she fought back — and wrote a book about it: Uplift: Secrets of the Sisterhood of Breast Cancer Survivors. Almost twenty-two years and twenty New York Times best-selling novels later, Barbara Delinsky is stronger than ever; and still donating all proceeds from the sale of Uplift to the Barbara Delinsky Foundation for Breast Cancer Research, which has funded twelve years of breast surgery fellowships at Massachusetts General Hospital.

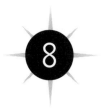

What to Do When the Boogeyman Doesn't Come

Barbara Delinsky

I expected to die of breast cancer — actually waited for it from the time I was sixteen and learned what had killed my mother. I was eight when she died. She was forty-five, way too young, but here I was at twenty and thirty getting college degrees, marrying and having kids, knowing — *knowing* — that I likely wouldn't live to see my kids grown.

Looking back, I see *survivor* written all over my life. I survived my mother's death, survived severe sibling rivalry, survived pudgy tween years and lonely high school years until I got to college and made friends. Breast cancer was a cloud following me wherever I went, but still I made the most of those years. There was something in me — something we didn't discuss in those days, but which I discuss now with friends all the time — something that drove me on. Being a survivor is an attitude. Is it inborn? I believe in nature far more than nurture, but in this case, I think it was a bit of both. Inner strength is like a muscle. The more we use it, the stronger it is. I was born with that strength, and my life demanded I hone it.

Then came breast cancer. Yes, I had known it was coming. I had my first child when I was twenty-four and doubted I would live to see him become an adult. Five years later, when I gave birth to twins, my greatest solace was that my three boys would have each other and their father when I was gone.

So there was no surprise when my doctor told me that the most recent cells she had biopsied showed cancer. I was running on a treadmill when she called with the news, and, rather than fall apart, I finished working out.

This is what survivors do.

My main sentiment, actually, was relief. After suffering all those years through mammograms and biopsies, after waiting by the phone in much the same way others with a family history wait, after marking my sons' every birthday with a little mental note that they were a year closer to being self-sufficient, I could finally act.

That first year, I had radiation, but a year later, when cancerous cells were found in the other breast, I had a bilateral mastectomy. For me, it was absolutely the right choice. I had waited and worried and feared for far too long. To rid myself of highly susceptible breast tissue was liberating.

Suddenly, *formally*, I was a survivor. In common parlance, that means I've been diagnosed with breast cancer and am still alive.

But, wait. *Still alive*? Is that all?

Hell, no. For me, it wasn't about being *still alive* but about having my life suddenly, richly, *lushly* open wide before me! That's what *liberated* means. For the first time in my grown-up life, that cloud over my head was gone. I could envision a future with my family, could see myself writing many more books than I already had, and imagined that I would die of something else entirely many years down the road — each shift in thinking a cause for celebration.

And celebrate I did, albeit in my very own way. I went on a Victoria's Secret shopping spree to buy bras to house my newly reconstructed breasts, bought a convertible ("Too dangerous," I used to say!), even got a tattoo. I began expressing my opinion more. My husband blamed that on menopause; I blamed it on a new boldness that came with beating breast cancer.

Through all this, no one outside of my immediate family knew I'd had breast cancer. Truly? I didn't want people asking me, sympathetically, how I was feeling. I didn't want a constant reminder. I'd had cancer and moved on.

Or had I? I'm a writer, and while I try to never write about people I know, personal experiences do creep in. I was, oh yes, *five years free* when a breast cancer survivor appeared in one of my books. I hadn't planned for that character to be a survivor. She just popped in and insisted on being heard. Her book, *Coast Road*, was a breakthrough book for me — my very first hardcover (of now twenty-two) to hit the *New York Times* list. My survivor, Katherine Evans, was a secondary character, but readers wrote me about her in droves. She was attractive, artistic, and upbeat. They saw her as a role model.

After two years of readers' letters, I knew what I had to do. Women wanted to hear about those who were surviving breast cancer, and, through my writing, I had a platform to bring them together. And so, *Uplift* was born. Formally titled *Uplift: Secrets from the Sisterhood of Breast Cancer Survivors*, it is a compilation of practical tips and upbeat anecdotes from survivors. I started with my own mailing list and word spread from there. Now, after four editions (each with new material), *Uplift* contains the words of more than 450 breast cancer survivors.

I only do book tours when a publisher puts a gun to my head. After *Uplift* was published, though, I agreed to speak at a survivors' dinner. I have to tell you, that first speech was a life-altering experience for me. The sheer energy of 1,200 women, all survivors, all strong and smiling and upbeat, was an inspiration. I've done other speeches since, and it's always the same. We survivors are a powerful group.

Uplift was first published in 2001. Fifteen years later, it is still one of a kind in the width and breadth of its contributors. I can't tell you how gratifying it is when a survivor tells me that *Uplift* helped her. And the success of the book goes beyond its readers. For all these many years, my proceeds from *Uplift* have funded a breast surgery fellowship at Massachusetts General Hospital. It just doesn't get any better than this!

Twenty years free now, I've often referred to "life ABC," life After Breast Cancer, and the letter analogy is correct. Surviving breast cancer was, for me, like starting at the beginning of the alphabet. My life opened up to new, different, better experiences.

Has it been all hunky-dory? Of course not. Radiated tissue doesn't reconstruct well, meaning that the chest wall on my left side protests every time I take a deep breath. These reconstructed breasts have settled into something not terribly pretty. I miss having a soft, sweet cleavage, miss the tingle of nipples, miss the nude beach on St. Bart's. I panic when each new little bump appears on my breasts, all perfectly harmless calcifications.

But I'm alive. My world is still bright, and I'm doing new and different things. My three sons are grown and married, I have three wonderful daughters-in-law and eight fabulous grandchildren. I took up tennis and am loving the camaraderie. I went off with eight strangers for an island adventure last fall. I'm reading more, taking the time to savor a brilliant novel. I'm still writing, but at my own pace.

Bottom line? I'm calling the shots. This, more than any other single fact, defines to me what being a survivor is about.

Breast cancer is an opportunity. This isn't an original thought. I actually cribbed it from a speech given by the father of a young cancer survivor — not even breast cancer — but the message is the same. Having any kind of cancer, any kind of life-threatening illness, is an opportunity to show what we're made of. We can either wither, cave in on ourselves, and resign ourselves to death, or we can reach out and fully embrace life.

Some say that if we cheat death we have a responsibility to make the most of life. I cannot disagree.

My mother died in 1954, at a time when early detection was nonexistent and treatment was barbarous. Back then, breast cancer was thought to be a woman's fault. Those who had it endured through their shame and pain in silence.

How far we've come!

MARISSA JARET WINOKUR danced her way into
the hearts of America as the fan-favorite on the hit ABC
series *Dancing With the Stars* during the sixth season. Marissa's
incredible personality and infectious smile won the fans' hearts,
and America voted for her over and over again, keeping her on
the show to the semi-finals. Currently, Marissa has recurring roles
on two television series: *Playing House* on USA and *Melissa and
Joey* on ABC Family. She was last seen on TV Land's *Retired at 35*,
starring opposite George Segal and Jessica Walter.

Marissa is perhaps best known for creating the role of Tracy
Turnblad in the hit Broadway musical *Hairspray*, a performance for
which she won a Tony Award, a Drama Desk Award, and an Outer
Critics Circle Award for Outstanding Actress.

A native of New York, Marissa started her career on the stage,
appearing as Jan in the Broadway production of *Grease*. After
moving to Los Angeles, Marissa quickly landed roles in the
features *Teaching Mrs. Tingle* and *Never Been Kissed*. These were
followed by her memorable roles in *Scary Movie* and *American
Beauty*. She also co-starred with Drew Barrymore and Jimmy
Fallon in the Farrelly Brothers' film *Fever Pitch*. On television,
Marissa has appeared on many shows, including *The Talk*, *Stacked*,
It Was One of Us, and *Dance Your Ass Off*. She starred alongside
Fran Drescher and Mark Consuelos in the ABC Family Channel
romantic comedy *Beautiful Girl*.

As a cancer survivor, Marissa works closely with Stand Up 2
Cancer and other cancer charities, raising money for research and
sharing the message that there is life after cancer. Marissa and
her husband, comedy writer Judah Miller, live in Los Angeles with
their son Zev.

Too Busy for Cancer

Marissa Jaret Winokur

As I think about being a cancer survivor, it seems incredible how *normal* my life is today.

This month (December 2015) marks my fifteenth year of being cancer-free! I was twenty-seven years old when I was diagnosed with cervical and uterine cancer. I think back and as weird as it sounds I am a bit grateful I was so young. In my twenties I was invincible and fearless. Nothing was gonna hold me back!!!

I had just started rehearsals for *Hairspray*, playing the lead in my first Broadway musical, and I refused to let cancer get in the way of my dreams. That attitude was invaluable. I was basically "too busy" for cancer! I was extremely proactive and never felt sorry for myself.

I kept my cancer a secret for fear of being fired from my job. In a way, I think the dual life "helped" me. I didn't have to talk about it with everyone; no one came at me with those "I'm so sorry eyes." I can honestly say I was able to live happily, being in denial. Healthy? Hell, no, but when I was informed I needed to have a radical hysterectomy (meaning my uterus and the cervix would be removed, but my ovaries would stay intact) I never thought about the consequences — I only thought: *Get this cancer out of me*!!! I wasn't thinking about not being able to carry a child I didn't know, I was thinking about myself and *living*! It sounds so selfish, now that I am a proud mom of a son, but that selfishness kicked cancer's ass.

After the surgery, I continued to live my life in denial. I opened in *Hairspray*, still not telling a soul what I had gone through. Even though I was healthy and knew I wouldn't be fired, I just didn't want the audience to know I was ever sick. I wanted them to love my character of Tracy Turnblad and not feel sorry for Marissa Winokur.

My secret was safe for many years. That was until I was happily married and wanted to have a child. That's when my missing uterus became a real problem. For the first time, five years after my radical hysterectomy, I felt like a cancer victim. I started feeling very sorry for myself. I was cancer-free, but cancer had stolen my chance of ever giving birth to a baby.

I finally began talking about my "cancer" but it was only in terms of not being able to have a baby! I was devastated — I always wanted a big family. I wasn't going to give up without a fight. I may have been thirty-three, but the twenty-something girl inside me came out swinging!! I was super proactive and knew I was meant to be a mom. I spent half my day learning about "how to get a surrogate" and the other half hiking Fryman Canyon, crying about wanting/*needing* to be a mom.

My husband and friends were very patient and helpful. They helped me understand that a lot of people have fertility problems and that's what this was: just another fertility problem. We were able to find a wonderfully caring, selfless woman to help us carry our son. The love of my life was born July 22, 2008 at 11:45 p.m., just making the cut-off by fifteen minutes for his astrology sign to be . . . you guessed it — *Cancer*. Yup, my son Zev has taken the curse off the word, he is a beautiful Cancer.

After Zev was born, I didn't waste much time thinking about my cancer. I never wanted it to define me. I thought of it as something from my past that was easy to forget. There was basically no reason to look back at this episode in my life. That was until a few months ago, when I received an e-mail from a dear friend who is a thirty-six-year-old mother. She had been diagnosed with breast cancer and was looking at a long road ahead.

As I read her note I began to cry, not pretty tearing up, but hysterical weeping. I cried for her, her daughter, her husband, her mom, and then I cried for myself. All of a sudden, it was as if fifteen years of denial came bubbling up to the surface. I felt like I was back in my little, one-room apartment, all alone as I found out I had cancer and would never be the same again. I cried for days. That's when I discovered something I had never really thought about before: that *I was a cancer survivor*. I was proud, and I didn't want to ignore that.

It was a defining moment in my life. It has made me who I am today. A fighter, a *survivor*. Knowing how my friend felt, I immediately asked her if we could get together. There was something I wanted to give her:

the piece of the puzzle that no one else had for her. I had the happy ending! I had the inside scoop on cancer. This was and is my advice to her and anyone else who needs it: Don't feel sorry for yourself. You are a fighter. You are a winner.

Surround yourself with a team that will help you to fight when you're feeling tired. When you have cancer, it can be a really shitty time. *It sucks, it's not fair.* But you didn't do anything wrong; this is just bad luck. You do not need to find a silver lining today. One day, years from now, you may be able to see the rainbow, *but fuck that today.* You are at war and you need to do everything you can to win this battle. You can cry later, but you don't have time for that now. This is the time for you to fight. Remember: *Fighters win.* YOU ARE THE STRONGEST PERSON I KNOW.

Today, the last thing on my to-do list, after dropping my son at baseball, is to drive across town to leave food at my friend's door. Today, she has her third round of chemo and a bunch of her friends have a "meal train" to make sure that she and her family are fed and stay strong these next few months. I know my store-bought soup won't make her better, but having a team behind her will. I know she can't see the sun behind the storm today. But I want her to know: Today, she is a warrior.

For me, fifteen years after my diagnosis and surgery, I can see the light. I am able to show other people that you can win. You can even sometimes forget you ever had cancer. Life will be the same someday or even better. My wonderful son Zev would never have been born if I hadn't had cancer when I was twenty-seven. I would have been a mom, I would have had a child, but I would not have had Zev. I am never sorry and I will never look back with sadness again about my cancer. It brought me Zev. He is the definition of a silver lining. I didn't know that when I was fighting for my life, but I know it now. I am proud to say I AM A CANCER SURVIVOR!

JENNIFER HAYDEN writes and draws original graphic
novels. Her newest book, *The Story of My Tits*, is a 352-page
memoir about her life and her experience with breast cancer.
It was named one of the best books of 2015 by the *New York
Times*, NPR, *Library Journal*, Amazon.com, *Paste*, *GQ*, *Mental Floss*,
and *Forbes*. Hayden's first book, the autobiographical collection
Underwire, was excerpted in *The Best American Comics of* 2013,
and her webcomic *S'Crapbook* earned a notable listing in *The
Best American Comics of* 2012. She currently posts the daily diary
strip *Rushes* at thegoddessrushes.blogspot.com and her work
has appeared in several print anthologies. She lives in Central
New Jersey with her husband, two cats, one very old dog, and
sometimes their two college-age children. Join her online at
www.jenniferhayden.com and goddesscomix.blogspot.com, on
Facebook at jenniferhaydenauthor and on Twitter @JenhayGoddess.

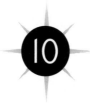

The Story of My Tits

Jennifer Hayden

(Editor's note: Every once in a while, a book comes along that breaks new ground, providing a wholly unique perspective that helps us understand a personal experience in fresh ways. Jennifer Hayden's universally acclaimed, graphic memoir The Story of My Tits is just such a book and I am pleased to share this brief excerpt from it with you.)

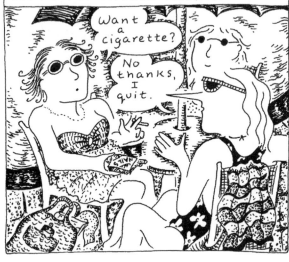

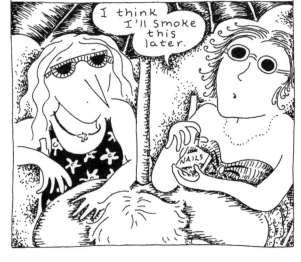

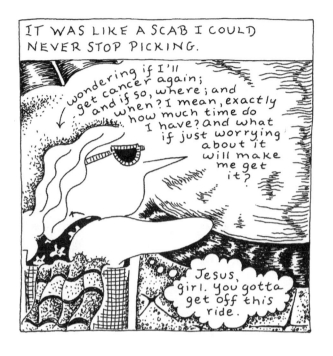

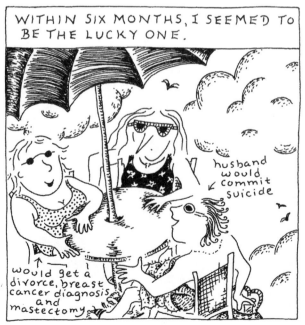

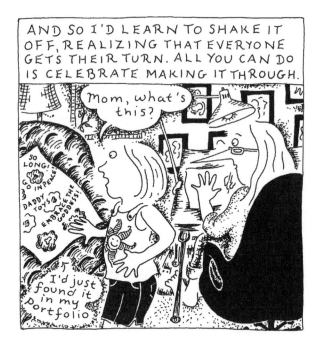

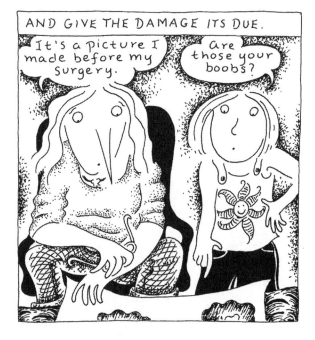

JENNIFER HAYDEN

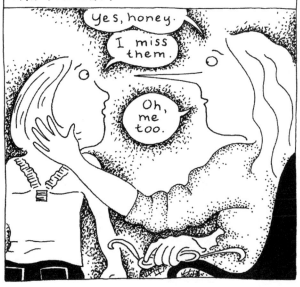

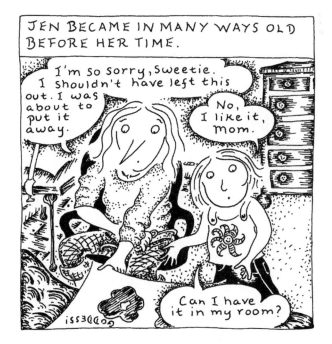

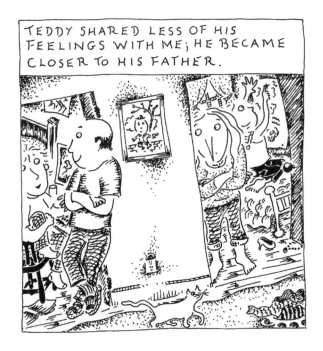

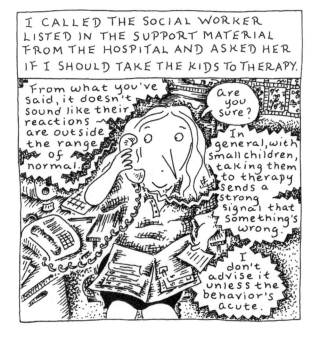

SO I DECIDED TO LET THEM HEAL THEMSELVES.

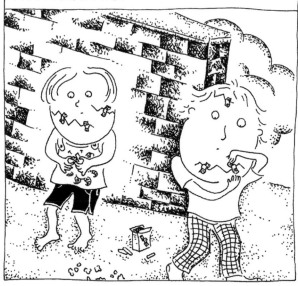

I ALSO TOOK MY ONCOLOGIST'S ADVICE AND GOT TESTED FOR THE BRCA GENE MUTATION ASSOCIATED WITH INHERITED BREAST AND OVARIAN CANCERS.

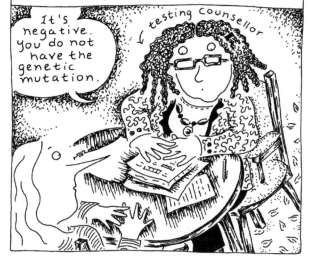

It's negative. You do not have the genetic mutation.

testing counsellor

N INA   R UBERTO , who was diagnosed with breast cancer
just two days after celebrating her fortieth birthday, is the proud
mother of three children: Hunter, Fierra, and her inspiring fifteen-
year-old daughter Capri Ruberto Anderson, who wrote the song
"Hope" at twelve years old while she watched Nina battle cancer.
Nina is an award-winning Canadian Realtor, businesswoman,
public speaker, and adventurer. She was born in the small
Canadian city of Thunder Bay and later left home to attend and
graduate from The University of Western Ontario. She has spoken
throughout Northwestern Ontario about her cancer story, and
since her recovery, has moved her family to Toronto, Ontario,
where she continues to work and support her children and their
big dreams.

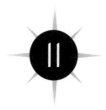

I Wore My Heels to Chemo

Nina Ruberto

"Happy 40th Birthday, Nina!!"

The banners were everywhere. I was surrounded by my husband, three children, family, and two hundred of my closest friends. It was a fabulous party, full of smiles, food, and dance. Everyone was celebrating my life, but do you know when you just have that uneasy gut feeling in the pit of your stomach? Yup. Two days later, I found myself sitting in my doctor's office, staring at a Kleenex box to the right of his shoulder as I heard the words "aggressive breast cancer" and I couldn't hear much more. . . . I just wanted the tissues in that box. I'm glad that I didn't know then the difficult journey I was about to embark on.

Like a zombie, and never taking my eyes off that Kleenex box, I asked the textbook questions through my tears: "Would I lose my hair?" "Did I have to take time off from work?" "Was I going to die?" Blankly, the doctor directed me to read a seven-hundred-page book that would answer all of my questions. *Are you fucking kidding me?* Left completely alone to navigate the coming months, my focus became my children and somehow getting mentally strong.

Nothing can really prepare you for the unknowns. Life got chaotic. I remember sitting in the driver's seat of my car and having to explain to my son and two daughters that I was going to start to look different. Mommy was going to lose her hair. I tried to make it exciting, like we would get to pick out fun, colorful wigs, but they knew what I was trying to do.

My youngest teared up, whispering, "But Mommy, you have the prettiest hair in the family." Oh, the moments. My cancer journey is filled to the rim with tear-jerking moments. I remember the day before my very first chemo treatment. I didn't want to go to sleep. I cleaned the house and reorganized my purses, and stared into the mirror — a lot. I knew that when I woke up, it would be the beginning of my physical transformation. I just didn't want the next day to come. I remember doing something very unusual. Before I closed my eyes, I took a smiling selfie. I wanted to remember what I looked like before the changes.

When the next day inevitably came, I made a promise to be positive. The warrior within me awoke. Instead of wearing my usual comfy sweats and sneakers, I put on a fantastic top, jeans, and my prettiest heels. I walked into that chemo unit like I was going out for a night on the town. I thought to myself, *I'm young, I'm strong and athletic, how bad could it be?*

I thought I had taken the first treatment quite well, but three hours after I got home, I was not able to move a single bone in my body. I could not even lift my arms or walk. So began sixteen weeks of nausea and weakness. Chemo sucked. I took it so badly and I'm not sure why it hit me so hard every time. I would wake up and keep repeating, "I am healthy" over and over again, hoping my body would transform and kill the cancer forever. I had to fight it daily, both mentally and physically. I had to do everything that I could.

The day my hair started to fall out was unforgettable. It was ten days after my first chemo treatment. I had dragged my butt out of bed to visit with my best friends. As I was trying to say something clever, I flicked my hair with my hand, and a bunch of my long black strands came out and hit the floor as if in slow motion. My girlfriends all stared at me in disbelief. No one knew how to react, and when I ran my other hand through the other side and another clump of hair was left in my hand, we all teared up at the same time.

My transformation into a visible cancer patient began. I shed for three days, and then after some coaxing, my brother came over to shave my head. My children each took turns cutting away. I wanted to make it fun for them. I don't know what was more difficult, hearing the clippers cut away my mane or watching my seventy-five-year-old mother stare at me with the saddest eyes I've ever seen.

Oddly enough, I got on the floor and collected my hair into a little baggie. I still have it. I just can't throw it out. It somehow represents something to me that is so monumental, yet so vain. It was like keeping a piece of something from someone that died, and every once in a while I grab the Ziplock bag and touch that old hair. It's almost bizarre. Looking back at those milestones, I remember feeling that breast cancer had stripped me of all the things that made me feel like a woman: my long black hair, eyebrows, eyelashes, my breasts, my nails . . . so, so cruel but I battled on as positively as possible. That warrior inside told me that I had to survive. I had to fight as hard as I could, and one day I would come back from this a better woman. I hoped.

Each of my three children dealt with watching me transform very differently. My son was very quiet, pretending not to notice anything but always telling me I was beautiful. My youngest daughter kept asking me if I was going to die, and my middle child, Capri, took to her creative musical side. One day, I was in my bed resting from a chemo treatment, and I heard her in the basement calling me to come down. I was so weak, but with Capri's help I made it downstairs. I'll never forget standing there, watching my twelve-year-old little girl pour her emotions out in song over the piano. I burst into tears. It was so painful for me to feel it through her young eyes.

Capri's song "Hope" then took our family through an insane journey. Her raw, sincere words almost knocked me over every time. The song took on a life of its own. It was played on YouTube in almost every country in the world. What was really amazing was that so many wonderful things happened on account of that innocent song that was just initially meant for me.

While I was going through my cancer treatments, which included a lumpectomy, chemotherapy, a skin-sparing double mastectomy, and radiation, the song's effect kept me distracted. I had to accompany Capri to radio and TV interviews, shows, and performances. It was wild, as if something beautiful came out of such a difficult and scary time.

The biggest blessing was receiving e-mails from all over the world, especially from children that were going through what Capri was going through. It was amazing how it had inspired so many people worldwide. It was such a beautiful thing and changed our lives completely. As I healed, I began to speak at events for the Canadian Cancer Society and local Cancer Center. Capri and I were a team. I would tell my story and then she would sing "Hope." The combination was very powerful, and it made us have even a deeper bond. My joy came from educating and inspiring others.

The string of events that happened post-cancer were really life-changing for our family. I finished treatments and tried to move on with my life (whatever that really means). I began to focus on what made me happy. Having cancer and battling it gave me the strength to do things I never thought were possible. When Capri got the opportunity to attend a specialized arts high school in Toronto, I leapt at the chance to support her. I picked up my family and left a successful career back in my home town to start from scratch in a large metropolis. I wanted to do something that scared the crap out of me. I wanted to do something that just pushed my limits and made no sense. I leapt, knowing the net would appear. It was a life-changing move that I never would have taken if I hadn't been rattled to the core by cancer.

I will say that now, I have never felt so ALIVE. My children are thriving, I am the happiest I have ever been, and I am grateful for every day. Having breast cancer, as scary as the process was and has been, has really been a gift. For the first time in my life, I feel as though I am living my authentic life. Do I fear it coming back? Of course. It's a fear we live with every day, but it's also a reminder that every waking day is precious, and to not be afraid to live. Choose happiness. Choose to be fearless. My body scars are a reminder of my crazy life, and I will continue to power forward as a stronger and better Nina. It's funny, I think God often answers prayers . . . you just might not like the path he chooses to get you there.

CAPRI RUBERTO ANDERSON is a child of many talents. At the young age of twelve, she dealt with watching her young mother battle her aggressive breast cancer by expressing herself through her songwriting. The song she wrote for her mother ended up on YouTube and touched the hearts of people around the world. She has been a young champion for raising money for cancer research through concerts, the sale of her song "Hope," and she has had the honor of being the main talent at many fundraising events. She even was invited to sing onstage with Nelly Furtado. Capri now attends a specialized arts high school in Toronto, where she double majors in both Music Theatre and Dance. She has also started her acting career and will be seen in the upcoming TV show *BackStage*. The world seems to be her oyster.

Hope Is by Our Side

Capri Ruberto Anderson

(Editor's note: When I contacted Nina Ruberto about contributing an essay to this book, she told me the moving story of the gift her daughter Capri had given her. At twelve years old, Capri wrote a song of comfort and love to help Nina get her through her cancer treatment. I asked if Capri would want to contribute an essay from her perspective to this book. Capri said yes, and it's my honor to share her essay with you.)

I am fifteen as I write this, but I was just twelve years old when I fearfully watched my young mother, Nina Ruberto, battle aggressive breast cancer. It was probably the worst thing I had experienced in my young life. I don't think I even fully knew what was going on.

Growing up, I always had a special bond with my mother. We were and still are extremely close. I remember so clearly the day I accidentally found out. I came home from school and there was my mom sitting at the kitchen table with her brothers and my grandparents. It was weird because she would normally still be working at this time and she was acting very odd. She looked so scared. I remember asking her if everything was all right and she told me it was. But I know my mom inside out so I knew something was up.

Being the curious twelve year old that I was, I secretly grabbed her phone when she got up to use the bathroom. I could hear her vomiting, and now I know it was from her fear. I took a peek at her messages and stumbled upon a text to her girlfriend saying, "It's breast cancer." I didn't even need to ask, I just knew she was talking about herself. I literally dropped the phone and ran up to my room bawling my eyes out. The only thing I could think was *Why God? Why her?* I couldn't imagine a life without my mom. She is my best friend. I was confused about what had to happen next. After a long conversation with my mom, I learned that chemo, surgeries, and radiation were on the way. I think everyone in my family dealt with the situation in different ways. I channeled my emotions through writing music. It was my place of peace and it comforted me. As time went on and my mom got more and more weak and sick, so many emotions were scrambling through my head and I just had to let them out. So at first I started to journal and I would write in this tiny diary every day about how I was feeling. Suddenly those words turned into lyrics, then into music, and then into one special song that I called "Hope."

I would usually come home after dance classes and run downstairs to our piano and sit there for hours. Just writing and writing. Finally, one day I ran up two flights of stairs and told my mom I had something very special to show her but that it was all the way in the basement. At the time, my mom could barely walk but she knew how much it would mean to me, so she managed to make her way down with my help. Then, I took my place at the piano and once I played the first two lines of my song, she just stood there sobbing. I didn't mean to upset her. I guess that she was so shocked that I could write such a moving piece. She told me she loved it so much and then we kind of just went on with the rest of our days, not really thinking too much about it.

Then, the following week, I had a vocal lesson and my mom told my vocal coach about the beautiful song I had written. So I sang it for her and she also started to bawl her eyes out. She then proceeded to say I should sing it at her Christmas recital. I was kind of hesitant at first because I never thought of anyone else ever hearing it, plus it was pretty personal. But after two weeks went by — bam — I was up onstage, and everyone in the audience was crying. We took a video and posted it to YouTube so my grandparents could see it.

Without us even thinking of sharing it with our friends, my vocal coach saw the video of that performance and posted the link to Facebook. From there it went viral, getting hits from around the world! It kind of turned this whole sad situation around. We got e-mails and letters from so many people going through the same thing, saying how inspiring I was to them. I was so surprised at how my song affected so many people. Soon after that, I was asked to be on radio, and then I was interviewed on the news. I was flown to California and even got to sing with Nelly Furtado! Crazy, right?

I'm just happy I was able to make my mom proud and create good memories out of a time that seemed so dark and scary. The fact that I was able to spread hope to so many other people and families made me have this great feeling of joy that I've never felt before. We tried hard as a family to stay positive through it all. Laughing was one thing we did every day! I gotta say, it was pretty funny when my mom had no hair and came out of the shower, twisting her "invisible" hair up in a towel and then taking a look at herself in the mirror. I remember asking her, "What are you doing?" She had forgotten she was bald!!! . . . and we laughed for hours. It's the best medicine, am I right?

My mom went through her cancer treatments like such a champion. She always made things fun for the kids and stayed so positive. She could have been depressed, but she always looked for the positive in everything. She showed us how to pick ourselves back up when we were down, and to never give up! In the end, this whole situation made us all stronger as individuals and as a family. I am so grateful to have inspired so many with my music too. You might have cancer but cancer doesn't have you, and remember that hope is always by your side! <3

"Hope"
by Capri

(Verse 1)
Mama's coming home real early
tears are running down her face
I could tell that her heart was bleeding
my strength came tumbling down
Fear froze in her open eyes
I just couldn't recognize her emotions quite before
I cried down to the floor
then she said

(Chorus)
"Hope is by our side
I will be all right
I won't leave you,
never leave you
I will find the strength
to make it all okay
I won't leave you,
never leave you"

(Verse 2)
Things started to change real soon
always tired, I felt like she was gone
into another world
lost and feeling so alone
She couldn't help when I needed her
not by choice, she'd never leave anyone
No matter what life decides to do
I will carry her
I will carry her through

CAPRI RUBERTO ANDERSON

(Chorus)
"Hope is by our side
I will be all right
I won't leave you,
never leave you
I will find the strength
to make it all okay
I won't leave you,
never leave you"

(Bridge)
Why did the bright side have to fade so soon
why did you put her, throw her in those shoes
was that the right right path right thing to do
three kids and husband left to lose
so much to lose oh

(Chorus)
"Hope is by our side
I will be all right
I won't leave you,
never leave you
I will find the strength
to make it all okay
I won't leave you,
never leave you"

(Verse 3)
Mama's coming home real early
a smile's dancing on her face
I could tell she had hope within her
I know it's going to be okay

New York Times best-selling author S H O N D A   S C H I L L I N G is the mother of an Asperger's Syndrome Child and wife of retired Boston Red Sox All-Star Curt Schilling. Her book, *The Best Kind of Different*, describes the story of her son Grant's struggle with Asperger's Syndrome and the heartbreaking and ultimately blissful journey she and her husband took to understanding this often misunderstood syndrome. Shonda is also a cancer survivor. Her public battle with malignant melanoma, the most deadly form of skin cancer, has been featured in a number of publications and on televisions shows, including *Good Morning America*. In 2002, Shonda created The Shade Foundation of America, an organization dedicated to eradicating melanoma through the education of children and the community in the prevention and detection of skin cancer and the promotion of sun safety. The foundation partnered with the Environmental Protection Agency to create SunWise, a program designed to help teachers raise sun safety awareness in children. Shonda and her husband Curt also work with the ALS Association to help find a cure for ALS, also known as Lou Gehrig's disease. Since 1992, they have donated and raised over $10 million for the association.

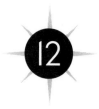

Life Is Filled with Curveballs

Shonda Schilling

I can remember the moment as if it were yesterday. "You have malignant melanoma." Now, fourteen years later, the memory is still crystal clear. I was a thirty-two-year-old mother with three children under the age of five. My husband Curt was in spring training. I called in and played the voice mail. "I need to see you first thing Monday morning" were the words the doctor had left on our voicemail. The kids had just hit their second wind that night and were still too young to recognize the panic that I am sure registered on my face.

I didn't want to bother the doctor if it was nothing. I guess this is what your mind does when you're frightened. So I called Curt instead, and told him the message. His reply was direct, and immediate: "I'll call right now." The phone rang not long after that. Can a phone-ring sound "ominous"? This one sure felt that way.

The next few days were a blur of doctors and that voice in my head that I bet every person diagnosed with cancer hears: *Why are you people going about your lives as if nothing is wrong?? I HAVE SKIN CANCER!* Then, I thought: *Maybe if I don't show fear or emotion, everyone will remain calm.* So that is what I did. The hardest part was after the kids had fallen asleep and I was lying next to Curt in bed. *What IF?* I asked myself every single night. That was hard. What helped me tremendously was my husband getting up every morning and making the two-hour drive to spring training and coming home after practice. He never had to say a word to me — it was just his presence that helped me through. Someone to whom I didn't have to pretend I was okay.

The hard part about getting cancer when I did was that we had just moved to Arizona and we knew almost no one. I relied heavily on my parents to babysit and help me with the five procedures. I wanted things to be normal. Going to the ballpark was normal for me. I could go to the ballpark and for three hours pretend that everything was fine. It was my escape from reality.

It took a few months for the story to get out in the press. By that time, I already had the routine down.

Removal, heal, and wait for the results. But the part I did NOT expect came next. I couldn't go to a game, the store, my kids' school, or even on an airplane that someone didn't come up to me and tell me that they had lost a loved one to melanoma and to please make sure I tell people how dangerous this was. Each story both scared me and broke my heart. I felt blessed to have caught mine early. But the thing so many people wanted was to give this a voice so their loved ones didn't die in vain. Give them a voice. Give melanoma a voice. It is NOT "just skin cancer."

This jump-started the healing process for me. When I decided to be that voice.

I wanted to put shade coverings up on windows at schools and I knew I needed to raise money. What I wanted most of all was to educate children. Within weeks I was contacted by the EPA, which had a complete teaching kit for sun safety and didn't know how to get it into the schools. The Arizona Department of Health had created an initiative but it appeared stalled, so we partnered. The timing was perfect. Sun safety immediately became a topic in schools and things snowballed on a national level from there. Out of this terrifying experience came the Shade Foundation, a nonprofit organization I founded with the purpose of eradicating skin cancer and melanoma through the education of children, parents, teachers, and the community throughout the United States. I believe I learned at the age of thirty-two that life is filled with lots of curveballs. We either let them strike us out, or we find a way to survive. I decided I was going to survive. One of the things that helped me most was choosing to share my story.

Parents told me, "My kids won't wear sunblock but since you taught them about sun safety they won't leave home without it." People who had lost family members to melanoma told me that friends would say to them that they didn't really understand what their loved ones had died of until they read my story. There were folks who walked up to me with tears in their eyes and said, "I have to thank you. I heard your message and I got checked. I had melanoma. You saved my life."

Since this happened to me I have been met with one life challenge after another. I chose to take the dark, scary, unpredictable times and try to find the positive. I find laughter and power in the unpredictability of life. Now, when life throws me one of those curveballs, I take my couple of minutes to cry, then I get up, dust myself off, and hit it head-on!

Known as the "other Dr. Ruth," RUTH HEIDRICH is a six-time Ironman Triathlon finisher, has held age-group records in every distance from 100-meter dashes to ultramarathons, the pentathlon, and triathlons, including eight gold medals in the Senior Olympics. She has completed sixty-seven marathons including Boston, New York, Moscow, and Honolulu, and has held three world fitness records in her age group at the famed Cooper Clinic in Dallas, Texas. She also was named one of the "Top Ten Fittest Women in North America" at age sixty-four. A graduate of UCLA, she holds a master's degree in Psychology, and a doctorate in Health Education. She has also lectured in this field at the University of Hawaii, Stanford University, and Cornell University. Author of *Senior Fitness*, A *Race for Life*, and *The* CHEF *Cook/Rawbook*, she has an "Ask Dr. Ruth" column on her Web site, www.RuthHeidrich.com.

Turning Breast Cancer Lemons into Lemonade

Ruth Heidrich, Ph.D.

I was a forty-seven-year-old marathoner, had been a runner for fourteen years, and believed I was as fit and healthy as I could possibly be! Talk about being on top of the world, I thought I had it all! My career was taking off as I was being groomed for a top senior executive position, my kids were successfully launched, and I loved the international travel that my job provided.

I'd studied nutrition in college and ate what I was told was a healthy diet with lots of chicken, fish, and low-fat dairy. I was in the best physical shape of my life; well, except for some arthritis, which I was told everybody gets by the time they're thirty. I'd started daily running at the age of thirty-three after coming across a book by the title *Aerobics* by

Kenneth Cooper, M.D. I read about all the advantages of aerobic exercise, decided to try to forestall the signs of aging that were starting to appear, and was amazed to find that I loved running! I found that I had more energy, I slept better, and, best of all, I could eat more and not gain weight. So, I had been running for fourteen years by the time I was forty-seven, and I had even entered races and run marathons.

What I didn't know was that my life was about to be dumped upon. In the shower that morning, I found a lump in my breast. I got right in to see a doctor who remarked, "Oh, I think you're probably too young for breast cancer." He did, however, order a mammogram, "Just to be sure," he said. The results were "negative," a false negative as it turned out, because I did have fibrocystic breast disease which hid the cancer. I was told to come back in six months. The next mammogram, the same result. This happened several more times. The third year, however, the lump was now the size of a golfball and very visible! The doctor looked shocked, took me by the elbow, escorted me down the hall, and said to the nurse, "Schedule this lady for an immediate biopsy."

This time the diagnosis was clear: Infiltrating Ductal Cancer, a moderately aggressive, invasive cancer that had already spread, which was indicated by more tests. There were thallium scans that showed "hot spots" in my bones, X-rays that revealed a tumor in my left lung, and blood tests that indicated elevated liver enzymes!

I was so stunned and disbelieving that I got second, third, and even a fourth opinion. Each doctor confirmed the findings, and as for my prognosis, none could tell me whether I had three months, three years, or what, just that it was "not good." They all recommended the standard chemotherapy and radiation. I could not believe my body betrayed me in such a manner! I was doing everything I was told to be healthy.

I was slated for chemotherapy; though I dreaded going down that path — I was terrified not to. I started searching for alternatives, any kind of help, anything — I did not want to die! That was when I found a little three-line newspaper item, "Wanted: Women with breast cancer to participate in cancer/ diet research study." I was sure that my diet, which even my oncologist called "healthy," had nothing to do with my breast cancer — so I thought I would help prove it. I ran to the phone and got right through to Dr. John McDougall. I was so surprised to be speaking directly to him that I started sputtering as I tried to tell him that I'd just been diagnosed with breast cancer. He said, "Get your medical records and come down to my office immediately."

At our first meeting, I heard him say, "Hmmm," as he looked over my lab results.

What now? I thought.

"You know, with cholesterol of 236, you are at as high a risk of dying of a heart attack as you are the cancer."

I was stunned by the deception of my body — cancer, arthritis, and, now, heart disease? I was a marathoner, for Pete's sake! These things can't happen to people like me! What was going on?

Dr. McDougall said, "Don't worry, all this can be reversed. Changing your diet will lower your cholesterol and with it, your risk of heart disease, and it will help reverse the cancer. And, to show that it was the diet that was responsible, there can't be any chemotherapy or radiation."

I was speechless! While I was processing all this totally baffling information, Dr. McDougall explained that he was conducting clinical research, which meant that there could be only one variable — the diet. If I had any other treatments, it would not be clear which aspect reversed the cancer. *Wait a minute*, I thought, *Change my diet or undergo chemo and radiation*? It was a no-brainer! "Okay, what do I do?" Dr. McDougall said, "It's simple — eliminate all animal foods and oils from your diet. Eat plant foods: fruits, vegetables, whole grains, and legumes."

I thought, I *can do this*! I already loved brown rice, whole-grain breads, and oatmeal. I just replaced the chicken, fish, and dairy with vegetables and fruit. No "transitioning" for me — I just became vegan!

When I returned to the oncologist and told him what I was doing, he scoffed and assured me that diet had nothing to do with my getting cancer. And yet, in a matter of weeks, the serious bone pain, that even narcotic medication could not relieve, had disappeared. The hot spots in my bones had significantly receded, and within three months, they were completely gone. The chest X-rays, to this day, still show an encapsulated tumor in my left lung, which hasn't grown in thirty-four years since my diagnosis, and my liver enzymes are now normal.

It was during all this turmoil that I happened to see the Ironman Triathlon on TV. I was awestruck! I leaned forward to get a closer look at what was unfolding and thought, *I've got to do that!* I saw the 2.4-mile swim, the 112-mile bike, and then the 26.2-mile marathon. I knew I could handle the marathon and naïvely thought just adding swimming and biking would be a piece of cake! Then it hit me: I'm now a cancer patient, and, besides, looking at all the young bodies, at forty-seven I'm way too old. But then I realized, what an opportunity I was being given: diet does affect cancer and I can show people that you can do one of the toughest races in the world on a vegan diet — and at a relatively advanced age to boot!

I added biking and swimming to my running. Training daily, I could see amazing progress in my speed and endurance. I also found that I was obsessing less about that awful diagnosis and appreciating the fact that I was really alive and that I was beating the cancer! What's more, I was enjoying my workouts and gaining confidence that I could attain one of the most ambitious goals I'd ever set for myself — to be an "Ironman"!

I did have to dig deep, however, as I was challenged like never before! Crossing that finish line of my first Ironman, I experienced a mix of joy, empowerment, exhilaration, and — total fatigue! I could not have gone another step!

Because of the history of osteoporosis on both sides of my family, I tracked my bone density over the next five years and found significant increases with each test, something I was told could never happen (in fact, I was informed that I should expect to *lose* bone density as I aged!). I was obviously getting enough calcium on this diet. My arthritis disappeared; my joints today not only are not arthritic, but I do my own daily triathlon as part of my regular training! My goal now, all these years later, is to maintain a high level of fitness and health. I'm now an eighty-year-old breast-cancer-thriver triathlete who turned cancerous lemons into Ironman lemonade!

BÁRBARA PADILLA is the vibrant, classical crossover soprano that dazzled the judges and the audience when she took center stage on *America's Got Talent*. Her spectacular performance of Charles Gounod's "Ave Maria," prompted judge Piers Morgan to declare, "It was the greatest single vocal performance we've ever had on *America's Got Talent!*" Bárbara's personal story as a cancer survivor resonated with viewers and her soaring vocals earned her first runner-up status, creating a devoted legion of fans worldwide. Her journey proved that she won't let anything stand in the way of pursuing her dreams.

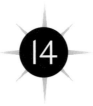

My Greatest Journey

Bárbara Padilla

Hello there! I am Bárbara Padilla, opera singer, daughter, wife, sister, mother, and friend. I have lived through real miracles that happened in my own flesh. Miracles that might be hard to believe. God has made me witness of His existence and has had real dialogues with this creature of His. Not because I deserve it, but because of My Creator's Will.

I was born in Guadalajara, Mexico, into a small, Catholic family: a single mom, a brother, and a sister (may she rest in peace). My mother, Luz, has always been a woman of faith. That same faith was passed down to us, her children, and has been very handy on many occasions.

Since I was a little girl, I loved music and had a real passion for the stage. For that reason I decided to study music and pursue a career as an opera singer. Yes, God gave me a voice and a good reason to use it: for His Glory. I enrolled in the school of music of the Universidad de Guadalajara and at the same time I obtained a degree in modern languages as a way to complement a career that would require them. Another reason was that I really wanted to know what I was singing in other languages!

I was in the middle of my many college occupations when I noticed a couple of unusual growths around my neck. For a while, I did not give them any importance because they did not hurt. I actually thought they were "muscles" that were being developed by my singing technique. Luckily, my mother was a social worker and the hospital where she worked was halfway between the school of music and my house. The bus that I rode to go home used to go right past my mom's office. One night, I just decided to stop and wait for my mom to finish her shift so we could have some tacos and go home together. Once in her office, I thought about asking if she could take me to see any doctor that might still be in the hospital so I could have my new and non-symmetrical growths examined. Thank God there was a magnificent surgeon who was in the building that night, Dr. Peña (RIP). He gladly examined me and after a few minutes, he said I needed further tests, but that the growths were definitely not "singing muscles," as I had called them. He did say that they did not look good and that they might be cancerous nodules.

No, I did not get scared . . . not then. I thought, *Hey, a few rounds of chemotherapy and I would be like new. . . . Or not . . .*

Well, after the biopsy and further tests, the results were not very promising. I was officially diagnosed with a Hodgkin Lymphoma (cancer) Stage IV (that means I was so dead).

I will never forget telling a good friend of mine about it, and she said: "Bárbara, God is great. And He'll heal you." But something about that statement was simply not right, and I said: "And if He doesn't, He's still great!" I really think that it is very important that we understand this. God's greatness does not depend on our healing, or anything at all. He is great, and if I had to die, everything was going to be okay. There was something else I knew: I had to fight.

The secret is simple: Take a deep breath and have hope. Yes, especially if the fight you're about to embark upon is a five-year battle. That's how long my fight took. And, of course, that confidence, hope, and faith were not always there. There were many times when I wanted to give up.

I thought I kind of had my life figured out, even after the diagnosis. But nothing prepared me for the most difficult part of all: depression. The chemical imbalances that I was going through provoked an interminable sadness. I broke up with my boyfriend; I lost my hair; I spent days, weeks, and even months in the hospital. Colors literally seemed dull because my eyes started to lose their ability see them. There was a time when my body lost all capacity to experience any kind of pleasure. I did not find solace in anything whatsoever.

Many times I thought about ending my life. Then I thought about what my first encounter with God would be. What would He ask me? Would He say: "What are you doing here? It wasn't your time yet. There was still a lot for you to accomplish." No, I did not want to find myself in that situation. So I prayed, and opened the Bible and there was always something. It was like being in the middle of the desert and when I felt that I was fainting, He gave me a sip of water, just enough to keep going.

What I did not know at the time was that God was building for me a new and wonderful life. He was preparing me to take a turn, and for that, it was absolutely necessary for me to be sick.

At one time, I decided to take a break from the treatments. Also, I decided to get a job. The State Choir of Jalisco was getting restructured and held auditions for singers and they were also looking for a new conductor. While I became the section leader and soloist, Dr. Harlan Snow (RIP) became the conductor.

After a couple of months, Dr. Snow noticed that there was something wrong with me. Of course, I had been avoiding going back to the hospital to hear what I already knew. I was having a relapse. Or more accurately, the illness had advanced. I gave Harlan the news and informed him of my decision: I was giving up.

Harlan and his wife, Joy, immediately started to put together a team of people that cooperated in diverse ways to send me to MD Anderson Cancer Center in

Houston. Needless to say, I did not have any desire to make that trip. However, I was grateful and decided to take the opportunity.

About a week before my trip, Dr. Snow had invited an important and renowned voice teacher from the United States to give a master class. After a long chat, he advised me to try to get in touch with a person he knew while I was in Houston. He gave me a name, I wrote it on a Post-It, and put it in the pocket of my jacket. Then I forgot about it.

When I arrived in Houston, Judi Hoover, who would be my hostess while I was there, was waiting for me at the airport. She had never heard me sing, but she knew that I was the soloist of Harlan's choir. She asked me if I wanted to sing for anybody while in Houston, to which I replied that I wasn't really prepared for that. I put my hand in my jacket pocket and I felt the note. I took it out, but there was only a name. No phone number, or anything else. Judi grabbed it and I forgot about the little piece of paper one more time.

The day of my appointment, we went to the hospital, and after some tests and procedures, I had some time before I needed to go see the doctor. We sat in the lobby and Judi stood up and left to make a couple of phone calls. About twenty minutes later, she came back with a smile on her face and said: "You have an audition with Peter Jacoby (the name on the piece of paper) tomorrow at 1:00 p.m. at the University of Houston." I later found out that he was the conductor of the opera of the Moores School of Music.

We saw the doctor who told me the same thing my doctors in Guadalajara had said: The lymphoma was way too advanced and I needed a bone marrow transplant. That was the end of the story with MD Anderson. I never went back there, nor did I see another doctor there. However, it was the beginning of the most amazing adventure of my life. The next day we went to see Peter, I sang, and he offered me a full scholarship to attend the music program. He was giving me the perfect reason to stay alive. But first, I had a long way to go.

I went back to Guadalajara. Doctors debated about the transplant; they said I was not a good candidate because of the damage caused by the number of treatments I had already received. At first they hoped that some more aggressive chemo rounds would do it. So, for the next year I underwent several more treatments. I had two more months before I had to go to Houston to start my music program. But the tests revealed a small tumor in the neck area. My medical team decided that the best way to go was radiation. One tiny detail: I was not going to be able to sing again. My world crumbled in that moment, and I thought I would have to reinvent my whole identity. My mother then said to me: "The doctors are not God, and you have to stay alive if you want to sing." And sure enough, God had His own plan. I underwent the radiotherapy and, miraculously, I never lost my voice.

I started the music program at the University of Houston in January of 2000. That summer I had another relapse. The worst of them all. The only solution was the bone marrow transplant. As I said earlier, I was not a candidate. But Dr. Gilberto Morgan, then head of the Oncology department, insisted that, even with the very high risk, a transplant was my only hope. I even signed a document in which I acknowledged that the risk was greater than my chances of survival. I thought I was going to die. But despite the many obstacles and complications I had to face, a real miracle happened: against all odds, the transplant worked!

I traveled back to Houston in January of 2001 completely cancer-free, and I never looked back.

I got married, I graduated with a master's degree, I adopted a child, I was runner-up on *America's Got Talent*, and now here I am, telling you my story!

Remember, at the end of the journey, the last day of your life, you want to say, "I did what I could," and not, "I could have done more."

God bless you!

FRAN DRESCHER received two Emmy Awards and two Golden Globe nominations for her portrayal as the lovable Miss Fine on the hit CBS series *The Nanny*, a show she also created, wrote, directed, and executive produced. Fran also starred in TV Land's sitcom *Happily Divorced*.

An accomplished film actress, Fran won *Esquire* magazine's Five Minute Oscar for her memorable performance in the mockumentary *This Is Spinal Tap*. She has co-starred in countless films throughout her career with the likes of Robin Williams, Dan Aykroyd, Tim Robbins, and Billy Crystal, and worked with such esteemed directors as Rob Reiner, Milos Forman, and Francis Ford Coppola. But she is most proud of her starring turn opposite Timothy Dalton in *The Beautician and the Beast*, a film she also executive produced. Onstage, Fran has had the privilege of performing in Ron Ribman's *Rug Merchants of Chaos* at The Pasadena Playhouse in Los Angeles, *The Exonerated* in New York City, Neil La Bute's *Some Girls*, and the New York production of Nora and Delia Ephron's *Love, Loss, and What I Wore*. Fran also performed in a special production of *Camelot* at the renowned Lincoln Center.

Fran is also an accomplished author. *Enter Whining*, her first book, was on the *New York Times* best-seller list. For her book, *Cancer Schmancer* (also a *New York Times* best-seller), she received the prestigious NCCS Writer's Award.

A uterine cancer survivor and leading health advocate, Fran is the President and visionary of the Cancer Schmancer Movement. She was instrumental in getting the United States' first Gynecologic Cancer Education and Awareness Act passed into law and was appointed to the distinguished position of Special Envoy for Women's Health Issues by the U.S. State Department.

Fran is the recipient of the John Wayne Institute Woman of Achievement Award, the Gilda Award, the City of Hope Woman of the Year Award, the Hebrew University Humanitarian Award, and the Albert Einstein College of Medicine's Spirit of Achievement Award, among many others.

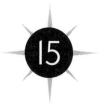

Cancer Schmancer

Fran Drescher

Both Elaine and Rachel said they wanted to be with me for the PET scan. Wednesday at four-thirty was the time; Nuclear Medicine was the place. John would arrive a bit later after a meeting he had. Camelia would pick me up and drive me to the hospital. Kathy would stay with Esther.

I must say, I was blessed to find myself surrounded by all these very wise and loving women. Each had known what it was to live life, as well as to feel pain and heartache. With them I can speak freely about hormones, cancer, and growing older. Without inhibition or embarrassment I can talk about my estrogen patch, gray hair, or wrinkles. They helped ease me into my new reality as painlessly and shamelessly as possible, pointing out the bumps in the road so I might fall fewer times and trip less. More and more I believe in a master plan and the subtle maneuvers from the angels above.

When Camelia came to pick me up for the PET scan, I kept procrastinating. I didn't want to go back to the hospital. I was afraid to take that test, afraid of what it might tell me. So while she sat with her car keys in hand, waiting, I felt the sudden need to prepare Kathryn a big bowl of spaghetti. I didn't want to believe this was anything more than a false alarm, but a tiny voice inside me feared the worst. I remember thinking, Is *this how it's going to be for me? Intermittent blocks of remission followed by one cancer after another?*

When we finally arrived at the hospital, the two of us navigated our way through the corridors to the dreaded door marked NUCLEAR MEDICINE. I was so grateful to Tom for squeezing me in that I'd brought him a box of chocolates. When Elaine and Rachel arrived, the whole atmosphere of the waiting room lifted. In two minutes we'd taken over and rearranged the whole lobby. Everyone was thirsty and I immediately began doling out cups from the water cooler. Always the hostess with the mostess.

Rachel helped me fill out the forms. It's so weird checking off the YES box for cancer, hysterectomy, appendectomy, and thyroiditis. I looked at her and said, "Can you believe this is me?" One of the questions they asked was whether I might be pregnant. My answer was no. By the time we got down to COMMENTS, all I could write was "Tom is nice."

It was Tom who took me to get the injection of the radioactive sugar solution. Rachel came along for support and also to use the bathroom. The framed posters, paintings, and photographs that lined the walls were the only memorable landmarks in a maze of otherwise nondescript hallways and doors. Both she and I made a pit stop at what Tom described as the "cleaner" bathroom, and then continued on to the room where I'd get my injection.

Tom said that I'd have to wait at least another thirty minutes to allow the stuff to spread throughout my body. I jokingly said I was going to start a rock band and call it "Radioactive Girl."

He also explained that a PET scan is particularly effective at photographing the lungs, since they normally won't take in the sugar at all. So Rachel and I returned to the waiting room, where Elaine sat knitting and chatting with Camelia.

Finally, at around 6 p.m., they led me in for the PET scan. The room itself was on the small side, and they felt only one person should sit with me in there. The rest of the brood sat just outside the curtain in the hallway, well within earshot.

Elaine sat with me initially and gabbed about her grandchildren while continuing to knit. She was a comforting presence as I hung on every word about little Ruby, the latest addition to the family. When John finally arrived, he took over for Elaine and filled me in on his meeting.

Through the curtain that divided us from Elaine, Rachel, and Camelia we collectively discussed where we should eat when this was done. After an hour of taking photos, I got dressed and we all walked over to Ubon, a Japanese noodle house. I kept my cell phone on as I waited for the call from my surgeon, who promised to give me an initial evaluation of the PET scan from the head doctor of Nuclear Medicine.

There we all were, drinking sake and digging our chopsticks into noodles and sushi, when the phone rang. We all froze. I flipped open the receiver as everyone looked on. Doctor #9 was so great about calling as quickly as she did. It was eight o'clock at night, and she was still making calls on my behalf. I wondered how many hours out of each day she actually devoted to her private life, but was grateful for her commitment to her patients.

The first thing she said was, "There's no sign of cancer anywhere," and I instantly gave everyone at the table the thumbs-up. In the morning she said she'd have a team of pulmonary (lung) specialists also look at the film, but that I should relax and enjoy my dinner.

When I hung up the phone, John, teary-eyed, thanked me for putting my thumb up so as not to prolong their agony. The first thing Elaine said was, "Call your folks and we'll hear whatever you tell them!"

My mom had been extremely anxious all day over this whole thing. Each time we spoke she'd answer the phone before the first ring finished, and this time was no different. It was 11 p.m. in Florida. "Yeah, hello," she answered, sounding a bit frantic — and rightfully so.

"It's definitely not cancer, there's no sign of cancer anywhere!" I said, rushing to get all the words out.

"Our prayers have been answered, that's all we wish for, that you should be well," my mom exclaimed. She sent her love to everyone, told us to enjoy our dinner, and added, "Now we can go to sleep." I was all aglow, both figuratively and literally. I raised my sake cup to my hero and heroines, and thanked them for their unending love and support.

PAMELA POST-FERRANTE, MEd, MFA, CAGS, is a cancer survivor, writer, teacher, and workshop leader. She created and taught Writing as a Therapeutic Modality in the Graduate School of Expressive Therapies at Lesley University (2003-2011). She leads Writing and Healing workshops for cancer survivors, and for those who work with them, privately and in Boston-area hospitals. She has the lead essay in *Living On the Margins: Women Writers on Breast Cancer* edited by Hilda Raz and published in 1999. Her essays and articles have appeared in books, magazines, and journals, and she has been heard many times on NPR, including two interviews on David Freudberg's *Humankind*: "Walking Through the Storm: What cancer survivors can teach us all about hope and quality of life," and "Living Fully with Illness," a joint interview with Susan Bauer-Wu. Pamela has been a guest blogger for a number of blogs, including Lahey Clinic, and she recently contributed prompts and instructions for a program of online writing at breastcancer.org. Pamela wrote *Writing & Healing: A Mindful Guide for Cancer Survivors* to offer to others the help she had not been able to find. The book was praised by Cokie Roberts, who said it "is a practical, yet beautiful how-to...[that gives] all the information anyone could possibly need to help those struggling with cancer express themselves by writing." It is the only book relating to cancer that was endorsed by James Pennebaker and John Evans in their 2014 book *Expressive Writing: Words that Heal*.

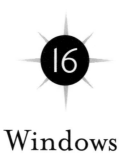

Windows

Pamela Post-Ferrante

Cancer changed my life. Not at first, with the initial two diagnoses, but because of the head-spinning years that followed, leaving a total of eight surgeries and two rounds of radiation between 1993 and 1998. There was also the destabilizing break-up of my twenty-five-year marriage, and the forced selling of my house in the same year as my final two surgeries. Losses piled up and up. In that first summer after the sale of my house, I found myself in a rented condominium with my two college-age children. I knew, even then, that much of the maiming came from anger, loss, abandonment, and being forced out of my home and community. These were the terrible aftershocks of the cancer. For, in the end, I was "cured" — the cancer cut from me.

Then, writing and community changed my life. I

had been accepted into an MFA in Writing Program before my first diagnosis. Radiation conflicted with that residency, but I was given an opportunity to participate in a nine-day meditation retreat. Mindfulness would be an important piece to add to writing, although at the time I didn't know it. Next came the surprise second diagnosis, again followed by surgery and radiation. The only way I could begin the MFA program was to double up on my last few radiation treatments. I didn't want to give up the chance for this residency again, so I made it through the intensified treatment schedule in time.

I drove to Vermont with a sense of freedom I hadn't felt in a long time. I knew that it usually never works to run away from pain, but this time it did. I had been writing in the cracks of my life for years. It took me thirteen years to create a short-story collection, which was finally with a literary agent, and for eleven years I had worked using therapeutic writing to help children with emotional and learning needs. I used creative writing techniques to initiate their writing. I would offer a "prompt," such as a picture, and say, "Write what is going on here. What's happening?" Or I'd give them an object and ask them to tell the story of the leaf or piece of old lace. Sometimes I gave them more of a help with the start by offering a partial first line: "I am Larry, a leaf and I...." The prompt usually helped them write about who they were and how they felt. Almost all did better both in school and in their lives.

I had measurable proof of how curative and life-giving it could be when the children tapped into their own creativity and used writing and sharing to release their feelings. But I never had experienced this for myself. Until the MFA residency, I had not had the luxury of simply writing or having a supportive community and advisor with whom to share the pieces I wrote. Each residency was ten days, filled with words and the healing act of "fully" listening.

In this first residency I was changing. Like a tapestry on a loom, the cancer years wove into the warp grey and muddy threads. The residency began to weave in the colors of golden light through creativity, release of words and stories, and safe sharing. I still use this light to find my way.

In the middle residency, I chose "Writing and Healing" as a critical thesis topic, using the same writing prompts that I had used with children and researching why this technique was capable of restoring self-esteem and healing old wounds. My topic was something most creative writing professors hadn't considered in 1995, but I found an advisor. As I wrote and researched, I felt embraced by the community; I felt safe and this saw me through the next four unexpected and more debilitating surgeries. When it was over, I had an MFA in Writing with a specialty in Writing and Healing. And I had a new husband.

I went back to working with children, but I couldn't forget what I really wanted to do: to help those with cancer. I found a program in a graduate school of expressive therapies (one of two in the country) within walking distance of my new home. I felt I needed more knowledge of the expressive arts and therapeutic practice. In the end, this advanced degree further grounded the sessions in healing for the body, mind, and spirit. Each session had a healing theme (Safe Place, Self-Care, Inner Healer, Gratitude, etc.) and a mindfulness meditation preceded the writing (initiated by prompts). We began sessions with a mindfulness meditation related to the healing theme and with the practice of following the breath all through it. Each session ended with a ritual (often a group poem) that provided important closure to the writing sessions. I began to lead the sessions in 2001 in hospitals and healing centers as well as in private practice. Halfway through the degree, a course I created was accepted by the Graduate School and I began to teach Writing as a Therapeutic Modality in 2003.

People who had known me before cancer wondered why I was setting aside my fiction. Logically, it seemed odd, but after all the stitches were healed and the drains removed, I knew I wanted to help those who were now out of cancer treatment and didn't know what to do next. I understood how they felt, and I wanted to offer the tools and format for healing on many levels that I was working so hard to create in the sessions. Leading them, as it turned out, continued to heal and shape me. I drew on who I already was and who I wanted to become to create the material for each session. As time went on, the sessions were offered to those still in treatment, their families, and caretakers.

It is now 2015. For at least a decade I have been struggling through fatigue that feels like walking into a strong wind each day. Some doctors offered labels of "chronic fatigue" or "chronic lyme"; rheumatologists and infectious disease specialists searched for other possibilities, always looking for cancer as well.

In 2012, an enlarged heart showed up on a chest X-ray which led to an echocardiogram, the use of ultrasound to look at my heart. I had fluid in the pericardial sac around my heart. The echo showed a small to moderate amount. They monitored it for a year, and then stopped the echoes in April of 2013, telling me that there was no reason to follow it further.

I couldn't teach graduate students Intensives because of exhaustion. When my book, *Writing & Healing: A Mindful Guide for Cancer Survivors* came out in December 2012, I stopped leading groups in hospitals and privately to concentrate whatever energy I had on marketing appearances, readings, lectures, magazine articles, and blogging. I walked away from all my best healing tools (expressive writing, creativity, community, themes of healing, sharing, deep listening) to name a few things that had been life-savers for me in the past. There was no marketing support for *Writing & Healing*, and had I been the healthy me, I could have managed. Now, I was staggering along trying to get the book known for the healing it could produce, all the while feeling that I was fading. Fortunately, I never stopped using mindfulness meditation. It was with me as I walked and went about daily tasks, and it carried me into sleep. The breath and the moment were always there helping me.

I was back at the hospital for an echocardiogram one and a half years from their letting me go. I brought myself in and told them I had more fluid around my heart. The level turned out to be moderate; in mid-November, they drained it to make sure it wasn't cancer. The fluid showed no carcinogenic cells, but they were highly irregular, as if they had been there a long time: evil and mutating. Then, as if awakened by the draining, the fluid began to climb, this time no matter what. In December's echo the fluid went up again in spite of medication. Another echo in January showed the highest level of fluid so far. When the cardiologist said he would schedule my next echo for sometime in mid to late February, I told him that would be too late. I stood up from my chair across from his desk and said, "So I will just fall over dead?"

"No," he said, without looking up. "You will faint first."

And that is the last I saw of him. I had a second opinion lined up. I knew I would be seeing another doctor.

In early February, during the start of an epic winter blizzard, I saw a cardiologist at a Boston hospital. After my appointment we walked to the scheduling office. She was able to get an MRI of my heart for the next day because someone had just cancelled. Without the doctor standing there beside me at that moment, I would probably have had to wait weeks or months for an appointment. The next morning I drove back to the hospital. I had the test and stayed for blood work. When I came home, there was an urgent message waiting for me on my answering machine: They wanted me to come back immediately for emergency surgery. I was told that my new cardiologist was arranging surgery for me, pulling together one team of cardiologists and another of thoracic surgeons as she was "driving away for vacation." (In fact, she was actually leaving for another job, but that wasn't public information at the time.) I had only known her for one day. It was a day that saved my life.

I was put on the cardiac floor in a huge room that looked as if it could be used for surgery, if needed. A wall of windows to my right gave me a view of snowy rooftops and roads. I loved the high views and the blowing, swirling snow. I felt as if I was riding the winds. "I am only half here," I wanted to say. A nurse ran in waving my book, excited that I had written it. *That's it for the book*, I thought. *I won't be able to market it any more.*

I was so sick by that time that I had almost no emotional reaction to what they would do to me next. The plan was to put in two drains. *Interesting*, I thought, remembering the roads in my neighborhood, which had been dug up in the fall to replace pipes and drains. *My body is like a road*, I thought. If that didn't work, they said they would put in a window and I couldn't imagine what a window in the road would do. Look into darkness? I had one foot in this world and one in another. My children had come. I had none of the worry and fear I had felt when going into surgeries at this very hospital almost twenty years before. I think I smiled and nodded. They looked worried.

And so, I had the two drains installed by the thoracic team, two of whom looked confusingly alike: young, tall, with short dark hair and thin, frameless glasses. I woke up at one point when they were doing the drains. I was in an upright position and I looked around and

I thought I was in a space ship. I saw monitors and cubicles in a circular position, and just when it got interesting I lapsed back into my drugged sleep.

The drains failed and I knew that, just like the street, they would dig me up again. This time it would be much harder and more serious. They would cut a postage-size opening in the pericardial sac so the fluid had an escape and my body would absorb it. They told me I could be in one of three places when I awoke: my bed where I was now, on the thoracic unit in case things needed watching, or the ICU. This was not multiple choice for me, so I didn't think about it.

I woke up in my room. I spent my time looking out the window. The snow drifted and lifted. Once, I saw my father and grandfather coming up the hill. Or at least I thought I saw them, as each was dead but dear to me.

It was a hard recovery, almost two weeks in the hospital, with two trips back to the emergency room with overnight stays.

After finally coming home, I slowly began to gain back my strength. I wore a heart monitor for a month, had many medications, and went back into the hospital to see the rheumatologist to figure out what had or was still causing the fluid.

It was the rheumatologist who told me a few months ago that it was the two rounds of radiation, both angles touching my heart, which had caused the pericarditis. My primary care physician said this was the consensus of all the doctors. So, I decided to pick up my book again. After all, it was created to help cancer survivors in or out of treatment. It could help those who have complications from the treatments as well. I should never have put aside my own healing.

Trying to promote a book is not like trying to heal (a body, mind, or spirit). Healing is quiet. Promotion is not. Stillness soothes. As I say in Writing & Healing, "The breath moves in the silence. Coming in. Going out. Softening the hard ground of your life." It is portable. When you are quiet and follow your breath you get beneath the surface of your busy mind.

I have picked up my book and plan to do some expressive writing from pictures (in newspapers and magazines and on the Internet) each day. I will tell the story I see in the photo or drawing. It will be a short writing of about five minutes (preceded by a brief time of following-the-breath to become still), and it will always have something to do with how I am feeling and what I need. In the quiet, your inner healer becomes alert as well. If you listen, it lets you know what you need. I return to the words I wrote for others and use them for myself: "Take your Inner Healer to a place where herons step soundlessly. Be so still that you hear a hush, a whisper, a kiss." This healing has existed forever; we have just forgotten how to rest in its arms. The book and I are not finished.

PATTI LuPONE swept the 2008 theater awards winning
the Tony, Drama Desk, and Outer Critics Circle Awards for Best
Actress in a Musical for her performance as Rose in the critically
acclaimed Broadway production of the classic musical *Gypsy*.
Patti has twice been nominated for an Emmy Award, has won
two Grammy awards, and has numerous film, television, and
on- and off-Broadway stage credits to her name. A five-time Tony
nominee and two-time winner, she was the first American actor
to win Britain's Olivier Award.

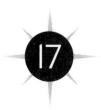

A Working Actor

Patti LuPone
with Digby Diehl

In the summer of 1999, Scott Wittman was approached by New York's Gay Men's Health Crisis to put together a benefit concert, which would become my solo Carnegie Hall debut. The two of us started brainstorming a new show with my musical director, the late and dearly missed Dick Gallagher. Jeff Richman would once again write the dialogue and the jokes. (He hates me calling them jokes. But there's no one better at writing them.)

That fall I was rehearsing the Carnegie Hall show, which was called *Coulda, Woulda, Shoulda*, in New York, and living a sweet life at home in Connecticut with my family. I cooked dinner, I did laundry, I attended my son's hockey games, and I had doctors' appointments. One was a routine mammogram.

I had the mammogram and waited in the office for the official dismissal — that everything looked good. I didn't wait long, and I didn't get the all-clear. A radiologist told me that there was a suspicious cluster of cells in my left breast and that I needed a more detailed mammogram to determine whether I had breast cancer or not. Apparently this cluster had been visible the year before, but now the radiologist felt it was time to do something. I asked why I hadn't been told the previous year about this abnormality. No answer or a lame one at best came out of his mouth.

Matt and I now started the rounds of interviews with breast surgeons and radiologists. We settled on a New York radiologist who believed there was nothing wrong with me, and we settled on a breast surgeon at Mass General in Boston in case there was. I went to New York and had the more detailed and excruciatingly painful mammogram. I continued rehearsing, with the concert looming just a mere week away.

Finally the concert was upon me. I was in the Parker Meridien hotel the day of the concert when I got a phone call from the radiologist with the bad news: I had breast cancer. She was sorry she had misled me, but she told me that I had the kind of cancer that, if I was to get breast cancer, was the kind to get. What a statement.

I heard every word she said, while in the back of my mind I was saying to myself, *I'm singing at Carnegie Hall tonight. Get to the point.* When I hung up the phone I was a total blank. Matt was with me and he figured out what was happening. We just looked at each other. What can you say at a time like that?

The phone rang again. It was Scott. I blurted out, "I have breast cancer."

He said, "You have a sound check."

It was perhaps the wisest thing to say. I went on with my life. I sang at Carnegie Hall that night without thinking of the cancer cells my body was now producing. There was no time. I went back to Connecticut, revisited Dr. Barbara Smith at Mass General, scheduled the operation, and had a lumpectomy, followed by six weeks of radiation treatments at the New Milford Hospital.

I was grateful that the cancer was caught early and that I had a great surgeon and radiologist. I am deeply grateful that I'm now ten years out, but it is never far from my mind that I could produce cancer cells again. I had a trainer at home who was well versed in what a woman should and should not eat during radiation. I lived on fish and soy. I viewed it as yet another test. There was no other way for me to process breast cancer.

The day I finished my last radiation treatment, I drove to New York City and started rehearsals for the New York Philharmonic production of *Sweeney Todd*. Finally I would sing my first Sondheim role, in an inspiring production that would be the third benchmark in my career.

With over thirty years of experience in show business, Emmy Award-winning makeup artist J A N   P I N G has worked on some of the most famous faces in Hollywood. The most memorable? "That's tough," Jan says. "Sean Connery, Howard Stern, Betty White . . . ," just to name a few. But Jan, a former actress and print model, says it took breast cancer for her to deeply understand the true meaning of beauty. That experience, which she describes as "endlessly profound," has changed her life forever. Since her diagnosis, Jan has been involved in many different organizations, helping to support women affected by breast cancer. She will be participating in the Tenth Annual Thrivers Cruise where she will do makeovers on ten deserving survivors. She currently works on Hallmark Channel's *The Home and Family Show*, continuing to add to her long list of experiences in television. In addition to working full time, Jan juggles writing, volunteering, and keynote speaking, discussing the emotional effects cancer treatment can have on self-image as well as the power of a positive perspective.

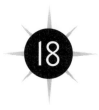

Strength in Sensitivity

Jan Ping

I am sensitive. I have always been sensitive.

I was told by a psychologist friend of mine that we are born with the five senses that are used both to help protect ourselves and make us aware. . . .

Well, I'm aware all right.

I can remember one time when I was a child, while my grandparents were babysitting me, I somehow got away with watching a terribly inappropriate show on television. I was so incredibly sensitive, and this show was apparently so upsetting, that I threw up my very exciting, not-normal-to-have-for-dinner McDonald's hamburger all over the living room floor. Now, thinking back to the early '60s, I'm not sure what show could have been upsetting enough to cause that kind of a reaction, but that just proves to you how sensitive I was.

Am . . .

But for some reason, I always thought of this sensitivity as my little secret. One that I needed to hide away as if it were something to be ashamed of. I guess my little acting job wasn't so great because it forced this secret of mine out into the open. People were always saying things like "Jeez, you are soooooo sensitive, toughen up!" It would catch me by surprise because I was certain that my "tough girl" performance was worthy of some kind of award.

To be perfectly honest, all of my greatest strengths in life are connected to this sensitivity and yet I am just now actually accepting and admitting it. Dare I say it out loud . . .?

I am sensitive. I have always been sensitive.

So, I am going along in this life of mine, being sensitive yet hiding it badly, all while trying to function day to day and pretending to be strong. Growing up, getting married, growing up more, having a child. Growing up even more, getting divorced, growing up more — again. Many heartbreaks, real and exaggerated, therapy off and on, classes, jobs, self-awareness seminars, meditation, life . . . and then cancer.

Hmmm . . . Did I just say cancer? Well, that wasn't part of the plan. Certainly not anything I ever thought I would experience. How is a "closet" sensitive girl supposed to handle this?

With strength, of course. Since I am *not* sensitive! I will just move forward with this new experience as if it were No. Big. Deal! I told my doctor to be aggressive with my treatment, and aggressive he was. His exact words were, "You are strong enough to handle it." And, unbeknownst to me, I was.

Even so, it was still kind of hard. Actually, it was *really* hard, and it constantly reminded me of my little secret that I wanted to keep to myself, all while putting on a brave face. I just wanted to keep my head down and get through it without bothering anyone along the way. I didn't want to be too much of an inconvenience (this coming from a very newbie strong girl).

I am sensitive. I have always been sensitive.

My treatment went very well. I had no complications to speak of, except the fact that I was battling cancer in the first place. However, during the whole process, an evolution happened. Nobody told me to expect this part. My nurses and doctors were so wonderful, explaining every medical step along the way, but they never once acknowledged that I'd experience deeper changes. I guess it could be because they were busy trying to save my life. Okay, I'll give them that one. They did a pretty damn good job. But these changes, these deep-to-the-core-of-your-being changes, were never mentioned.

For those experiencing cancer, let me try and explain: These changes can manifest themselves in many different ways. When you find out you have cancer you have to redefine how you see yourself. Your idea of beauty, the one that has been instilled in us from day one, *has* to change. Cancer forces us to accept the often permanent changes in our physical body and recognize our true beauty. Regardless of how much mental planning you do, nothing will prepare you for the moment you see your now-unrecognizable self. Your personal definition of beauty, of health, and of your own mortality all come into play at that moment when you confront your fears and choose to look at it all differently.

But guess what? There is something waiting for you at the end of a very long road. Like digging for buried treasure . . . and actually finding one.

Now, please don't misunderstand me, cancer is not fun. However, your outlook on the experience and what you choose to do with it is entirely up to you. I decided to make it a prize, an accomplishment, and it is my blessing.

Since this whole cancer thing happened to me, I've had the opportunity to do many things I never would have done if I hadn't had cancer. Seriously amazing things. Things my loved ones are proud of. Things that *I'm* proud of. Sensitive things. Strong things.

I can now say that I am:

A Survivor.

A Keynote Speaker.

A Published Writer.

A Spokesperson.

A Cancer Beauty Expert.

A Thriver.

Now, this growth took a bit of time. My "fabulousness" didn't just happen overnight. No, it was a process, one that I wouldn't change for anything. If you asked me even halfway down this road of self-discovery if I would be doing any of this, I would have thought you were nutty. And yet it all happened.

As a professional makeup artist, I've had the opportunity to touch and be touched by many different women all sharing the same life experience, connecting at a level so deep it sometimes takes my breath away. The fear, the pain, the changes . . . all disorienting. But only from this place of surrender are we able to find our balance. That's where the magic lies. When you find yourself in this place, your life can change. And other lives, too.

The evolution of my cancer experience taught me the amazing pleasure of witnessing countless women rediscovering their honest beauty. This insight comes slowly. The long, quiet, personal road you travel on can be both confusing and inspiring. The flashes of "Oh, this is what it's about" come in calming waves that leave you feeling as if all your conflicting emotions have finally been resolved. You go deeper and deeper until you reach that quiet place, and that sweet spot leaves a smile on your face. You have arrived. You have found your balance between sensitivity and strength.

I am sensitive. I have *always* been sensitive.

Okay, so I've admitted this out loud. Now what? Well, this secret of mine has given me a lot. I feel things. Lots of things. When a woman who has gone through breast cancer sits in my makeup chair, I feel her doubts, I feel her insecurities, her loss, and her struggles. Her body has just put her through this very demanding experience and now things have changed. Changed, in my opinion, for the better, although it may not feel this way to her. I've been there. It feels foreign and uncharted, like meeting a stranger that seems worthy of friendship but you're not sure. It just all feels so *new*. Is this woman in the mirror nice? Is she kind? Will she be there when I need her? Will she like me back? Will she *love* me back? Ah, there it is . . . it's always a bit scary allowing yourself to be fully engaged in a new relationship, even with yourself.

She has to get to know this new body like getting to know that new friend. But it takes time to do this. If the friendship is a worthy venture, she just might fall in love, and this is key. She needs to fall in love with this new friend because they will be friends forever. This new connection must be nurtured and cared for like a precious moment; unforgettable.

When I have had the chance to do makeup on someone going through cancer treatment, the opportunity to connect at a deeper level is possible. I explain to them that I have also gone through something similar, and immediately everything shifts. It calms. This newfound camaraderie is very powerful. Typically, these people start out in my chair coming from this uncomfortable place of insecurity. Doubting oneself physically is such a personal and private concern, and a lot of times people feel isolated and even embarrassed, thinking that they were "better" before cancer and treatment forced these physical changes. Well, having gone through this process myself, I have this to say about it. Treatment is vital. However, how we feel about our self-image is *also* vitally important. It can affect our mood, our energy, and even our will to move forward into a healthy, happy future.

When I am finished with their makeup and we both look in the mirror together, I literally can see the shift happen. It's a twinkle in their eyes, one of recognition of something new. Of their inner beauty.

They typically say that they look beautiful, as if realizing this for the first time. Or they say that they look like their old selves, only better. Sometimes they tear up. It may even be too difficult for them to openly acknowledge how they are feeling at that moment, but they will say something to me later. I was actually sent a note one time stating this fact after someone had left my chair because it was just too much for them to comprehend in that moment.

This reaction happens across the board, and it is an absolute pleasure to watch this new love affair unfold in front of me. Once you have seen this shift you can no longer deny its existence. It is just that magical and profound.

Reverting back to this secret of mine, the one I am now shouting out loud, I see that it has always been my strength. I just didn't know it, or didn't know how to use it. But this cancer experience has helped me to fine-tune my strengths. This scary, challenging process has forced me to get in touch with *me*. It forced me to look at myself honestly and get to know this new me from a different perspective. A deeper perspective. And guess what? I fell in love. Yikes, that sounds goofy, almost embarrassing. Almost, but not really. It actually feels like it's where I am supposed to be.

Sometimes things fall into our laps gently and other times we trip over the large obstacles right in our path. My cancer was one of these obstacles, and I nearly lost my balance. But in the last ten years, I've perfected my step. I've exercised, practiced, and actively participated in my life. *Everything* in my life now is deep, wiser. I have become best friends with that woman in the mirror, this new me.

So this is why I call my cancer experience a gift. Now, I'm aware that this is a bold statement, one that not everyone agrees with, but it's how I choose to look at it. And for me it really has been true. It has given me insight that I didn't have before. I have made amazing new friends, and I have also felt the deep heartbreak of losing some of those friends. I have grown, and I have achieved things I would have never achieved before. I have become strong — no, strongER. I am fully committed to this strength and for me it took this experience to get me there. My cancer journey allowed me the permission to embrace this depth of soul and to fully love and accept myself.

I am sensitive.

I have *always* been sensitive.

I am strong.

I *will always* be strong.

I *am both*, and this is a very good thing.

ELANA ROSENBAUM, MS, MSW, LICSW, is a leader in the clinical application of mindfulness meditation to cancer care. She has authored *Being Well (even when you're sick): Mindfulness Practices for People Living with Cancer and Other Illnesses* and *Here for Now: Living Well with Cancer Through Mindfulness*, the basis of many workshops and CDs with guided meditations. In 1995 she was diagnosed with non-Hodgkin lymphoma and subsequently underwent stem-cell transplantation. Her ability to thrive and embody mindfulness in the face of adversity led to the development of a mindfulness-based intervention for bone marrow transplant patients at the University of Massachusetts Medical Center, Emory University, and Dana Farber Cancer Institute. She is adjunct faculty at the renowned Stress Reduction Clinic at the University of Massachusetts Medical School where she worked directly with Jon Kabat-Zinn as one of the founding teachers. She's been teaching and educating patients and health-care professionals in mindfulness, including leading cancer centers, for over twenty-five years. Elana has a private practice in psychotherapy in Worcester, Massachusetts and is a sought-after teacher, speaker, workshop leader, and research consultant.

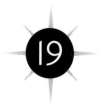

Living Well with Cancer

Elana Rosenbaum

It has been many years since I was diagnosed with cancer. I know because I count them. It was 1995 when I was diagnosed with non-Hodgkin lymphoma and it was a shock. I teach meditation and mindfulness-based stress reduction (MBSR) and this wasn't supposed to happen. The theory being that if you meditated, ate right, exercised, and had meaningful relationships you'd stay well. This is true but well does not mean being free of illness, loss, or death. It does mean that your relationship to illness, loss, and death can be altered in a way that relieves suffering. Attitude makes a difference. It is possible to be sick and to be well, and when I was diagnosed I set my intention to live what I taught in MBSR, which is:

There is more right with you than wrong.

You don't have to suffer.

Doing this is not automatic; unless you are born with a lot of joy juice or have a nature to see the glass half full rather than half empty, it takes patience, trust, and determination.

My father died of cancer, mesothelioma, a few months before I learned that I had cancer. I remember feeling happy that I didn't have to give him this news and I could spare both him and my mother worry. Mom never smoked but died of lung cancer at the age of seventy. This was ten years before I was diagnosed. I remember her being scared and how I used to comfort her sitting by her bed and guiding her in meditations to allay her fears. I recorded the meditations and left them with her to listen to when she felt alone and afraid. Being with her and allowing my words to flow breath by breath helped to calm me as well as my mother. The words were not as important as the love that was communicated between us. As I sat quietly with her, matching my breathing to hers, I felt the connection deepen between us. I did not know that years later, when I lay in bed in the hospital barely able to breathe, the presence of loved ones nonverbally communicating love and care would help me feel loved and held.

After my father was diagnosed with cancer, he lived independently at first and then when he could no longer care for himself he came to live with my husband and me. Rather than give in to sadness and regret at having to leave his home of eighty years, he saw cancer and dying as "an adventure" and would tell me, "You can't know what's on the other side unless you leave the shore."

Until his last breath, Dad celebrated being alive and always managed to find something to appreciate, even when he was in pain. He was grateful for the care he received, for his doctor, for a hot bowl of soup, or a coupon from the newspaper that he could cut out and give to us. He lived with us in a room next to the kitchen and each morning as I'd come into the kitchen he'd call, "Elana, Elana" until I went into his bedroom and with a big smile on his face he'd exclaim joyfully, "I'm still here!"

Mindfulness-based stress reduction, which I've taught since 1984, is about being here in this moment with all of our senses. The instruction is to bring awareness to this moment and when attention wanders, which it will, to escort it gently back to here, now. This takes practice as well as kindness and compassion.

Repetition helps as does remembering why it's useful to stay awake and be here — to be fully alive as long as we are alive and to be open to all the wonder of life: the happiness and the pain, the sorrow and the joy. As I tell my classes, quoting Thoreau in *Walden*, "Only that day dawns to which we are awake."

Intention is powerful and my intention not to suffer helped me to be well even while I faced chemo, subsequent stem-cell transplant, and recurrences. Again and again I brought my attention back to "here," to the fullness of each moment. I couldn't concentrate but I could feel a friend's smile. I could look out the window and watch clouds moving through the sky. I could focus on the possible and appreciate the comfort of a warm blanket and the coolness of an ice chip soothing the sores in my mouth or the potency of a gentle touch.

Now, I sit with others, some with cancer, others who experience the stresses inherent in living life, and I teach them how to be mindful and kind to themselves. I live with uncertainty. I am currently in remission but I still have cancer and have had a few recurrences. I can and most likely will have another, for that's the nature of this disease, but

I'm here now. How wonderful! I value each moment and meeting what it brings. *"Yes to life and all that's in it"* is my motto — even when there is a challenge, a disappointment, or a loss. Knowing that I can have another recurrence helps me remember to be awake and not take for granted the rising of another dawn or the extraordinariness of the ordinary. It helps me be open to what I feel and gives me the courage to try new things and no longer pretend to be what I am not in order to conform or be accepted. This gives me permission to speak my truth, which is very freeing.

It's wonderful to have energy. I don't take it for granted. There are times when this is impossible and the ability to surrender — to take a nap and rest — is a gift, as is the wisdom to stop and not push more than is needed. I've discovered that the more I can acknowledge my limitations, like getting tired more easily, the freer I am. When I am fatigued I don't think well, so I've learned to say, "Not now" not only to others but to myself. It's humbling to acknowledge I can't do something that used to be easy but what a relief. It helps me focus on what is possible . . . and a reminder to be grateful for what is available to me. I savor my vitality and do not put off what I think is important — like being with family and friends. Facing death helps me appreciate life.

When I was very weak and recovering from my stem-cell transplant, there was little I could do. I'd often sit on the sofa in our home, find a spot in the sunlight, follow my breath, and gaze out the window for perspective. I was inspired to write a credo, which I included in my book *Here for Now: Living Well with Cancer Through Mindfulness*. I recently reread the words and I found that they still apply:

Some people after a great battle go on to the next one while others choose to go home to rest and recuperate until they must fight again. I choose to fight only battles of mind that hinder clarity and wisdom . . . I shall use my experience to remember the preciousness of life and the gifts I have received. I shall challenge myself to live wisely and make meaning of my experience, letting it transform me. I shall work to bring peace to others, so they too, may be free. I am filled with gratitude to all who have helped me be alive and well. May I never forget the grace that has been bestowed upon me.

Many years have passed since I wrote this credo. I am now older than my mother was when she died but younger than my father. I continue to be aware of the timelessness of the present moment and how everything is transitory. I often *S.T.O.P.*: stop, take a breath, observe what is here and open myself to the full range of my experience, thoughts, feelings, emotions, and sensations, and then proceed. This helps me maintain perspective, cope with the difficult, and savor the wonder of life. There is so much to appreciate each day, sunlight and laughter, friendship and love. Breath by breath I acknowledge I am still here . . . and say thank you.

ENID SHAPIRO, MSW, ACSW, LICSW, is a retired clinical social worker who has had a fifty-year career working with families and their adult children. A graduate of Boston University and the Simmons College School of Social Work, Enid serves on a number of professional and community committees. She has been living with breast cancer for the past twenty-seven years. Enid is the mother of three adult children, has eight grandchildren, and recently became a great grandmother. She lives in Brookline, Massachusetts.

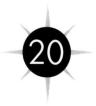

Attitude & Identity

Enid Shapiro

At ninety, it does seem important to reflect on how my attitude and identity have shaped my life and the way I have coped with breast cancer.

Diagnosed twenty-seven years ago with breast cancer, what I recall was my very first question for my oncologist: "How are we going to treat this?" It just never occurred to me to think that there would *not* be any way to deal with the disease. In retrospect, I realize my question represented the way I looked at the world in every aspect of my life.

At that pivotal moment I was in my mid-fifties, had three adult children, a responsible professional social work position, and the good fortune to have a very supportive husband, eleven years older than myself. He was possibly more shaken by my diagnosis than

I was. His first words were, "I never expected this to happen to us." He was clearly frightened. Once I learned the treatment options, my very first thought was that I had to tell my children — and in person — so they could see how I was coping and ask any questions. I wanted to put their minds at ease. My parental style had always been, if possible, to model by example the way to manage problems.

Was I depressed? Perhaps somewhat, but not frightened. I felt absolutely confident that there would be positive treatment options, and I just knew that my medical team would prevail. Now, thinking back, I truly believe that attitude absolutely played a major role in my personal medical journey.

How did I develop this positive attitude? Possibly, it was the environment in which I was raised and my early family experience. Years of personal therapy has never quite helped identify where it all started (i.e., experiences? genetic disposition? my DNA?). We are only just beginning to understand how personality and attitude develop. I believe it has been the motivating force that has helped me cope so successfully with multiple recurrences of this breast cancer diagnosis and treatment.

Have I allowed those experiences to determine my identity? Cancer has never taken over my life. Certainly there have been continual medical visits, at times cosmetic concerns (I did lose my hair at one point), periods when I felt fairly ill, but it has never been what I felt were the overriding issues in my life.

What are those issues? Social Justice and activism to "repair the world" have been what I view as a personal challenge. My Jewish heritage and the study of my faith have determined my identity. They most likely have been the motivating forces in directing my professional career and have kept me focused in the way I have been able to literally manage the emotional dimension of coping with breast cancer.

It has been my good fortune to have an extraordinary medical team at Beth Israel Deaconess Medical Center in Boston, Massachusetts. Physicians (there have been many) have played a vital role. My friendships with several younger women have provided the support that has restored me when I needed a boost.

Fortunately, I have always been physically active. I was endowed with a great amount of energy and needed to use it in a focused way. I was a pretty compulsive housekeeper and accustomed to doing most of my own housework. From a very young age, I was a swimmer and a skater, and I rode a bicycle; I spent several hours every day exercising in some way.

My father died at fifty-nine after nine years of illness marked by lung cancer, which kept him hospitalized for the last six years of his life.

I literally grew up with illness and it certainly played a role in the way I have approached my own brush with disease.

I met my late husband Mel at a political rally (his younger sister introduced us) and we were married in August of 1947, after a somewhat whirlwind relationship. He had only recently been discharged from the United States Army after serving for six years, two in the Asian theater during World War II. Mel was eager to settle down and have a family.

Given our backgrounds, we did establish a traditional Jewish family with the expectation that Mel would work and I would "keep house." Those were the beginning years of the women's movement, which lit a spark in me and fueled my own desire to give back to society.

Although I had three young children and a very busy family life, the recognition that I did not have a way to fulfill my life after my children left home was a concern. I needed something else. Energetic, very fit, and with the support of my husband, I went back to school. I was accepted part-time at the Simmons College School of Social Work and it changed my life. It took six years for me to graduate and get my social work degree, years that were marked by a very hectic schedule with very little time for reflection.

I grew up in a Jewish household and although I did not attend religious school, I understood that I had a responsibility to make a contribution to better the world. In Judaism, it is called "Tikun Olam," repair the world. Busy with a young, very active family, I always found time to volunteer particularly in the political arena. But I constantly felt a need to do more.

The years I spent in school, coupled with activities in my community, confirmed my desire to participate. I began to really understand the needs of others, the breakdown in public policy and education, and the importance of each individual contributing to society. My first part-time job experience in a hospital setting directed my career.

During my six years at Simmons, I had two yearlong field placements; the first in the Roxbury, Massachusetts office of Jewish Family and Children's Service and the second in the orthopedic service at Massachusetts General Hospital. Both were extraordinary learning opportunities.

My first job was at Beth Israel Hospital (now Beth Israel Deaconess Medical Center), doing outreach in a Jewish Senior Center in Chelsea, Massachusetts. There I developed a real thirst for understanding the history and experience of the immigrant population, both in their adjustment to their new country and their commitment to their Jewish heritage. After over a year, I moved on to a position as the Home Care Social Worker at the hospital where I was exposed to the changing needs of a burgeoning population of older people. Simultaneously, I joined the Massachusetts Chapter of the National Association of Social Workers.

My commitment to older people, a desire to do something to better the world, combined with some Jewish perspectives on social justice, directed me. Life seemed to be moving at a predictable pace when I was diagnosed with breast cancer. To say the least, it should have put a hold on all my activities.

But then attitude and identity played their important role. I talked with my physician and never missed a beat.

My first bout involved a radiation implant and necessary hospitalization. Those days I was confined in isolation for three days. Then came the follow up. I went back to work and began a routine of regular physician visits, constant blood work, and subsequent radiation treatments. Somehow, I plugged these visits into my usual routine. I also found time to resume my biblical studies.

Now looking back, I realize what kept me going was my attitude and how I related to the world. There were never moments when I felt I would not be cared for. I joined a group of breast cancer survivors and began to work to help other women make necessary decisions regarding their treatment plans. Everyone was different; each woman needed to think about her individual situation. Breast cancer is not a diagnosis of "one size fits all" dimension.

There was also an opportunity to help the organization Silent Spring explore how the environment contributes to the incidence of breast cancer. Now, twenty years later, it is beginning to identify where there may be connections. The federal government is starting to recognize this possibility. When I was diagnosed in 1988, The Genome Project was in its infancy, but constant observation was the way to understand what was happening to each person. Where was it important to put our energy? How did the political situation affect the allocation of resources? Was there a way to raise funds to create further awareness? How could we mobilize a cohort of citizens to do the work that was necessary to end this disease?

All of this actually fit in the pattern of the way I wanted to live my life. I became an advocate, politically believing that the federal government had a major role in contributing to the matter of breast cancer treatment and subsequent cure.

I hold that belief to this day and continue to support and work with the National Breast Cancer Coalition.

Now experiencing yet another recurrence I will be involved once more in a treatment plan. My physicians continue to have hope and I believe them. I have never let the breast cancer diagnosis characterize my identity and I absolutely will not let it do so at this late age. My positive attitude and my beliefs inspire me every day.

My religious tradition has not dictated specific answers to major questions, but rather provided values to be applied to life. We are demanded to involve ourselves in the task of building a better world. One of those tasks is certainly the treatment of disease and finding a cure for breast cancer. My attitude that we can, if we muster all our energies, find that cure, has enabled me to survive to ninety. Attitude and Identity have certainly played a major role. I continue to be treated for "metastatic breast cancer" but also have a great deal of hope that we will find a cure, perhaps even in my lifetime.

CYNTHIA THOMPSON holds an MFA in Sculpture
from the School of the Museum of Fine Arts, Boston, as well
as a BFA in Sculpture and a BA in Education from Colorado
State University. She taught art in public high schools in
Massachusetts, and attended Rochester Institute of Technology,
before returning for MFA studies, where her work migrated from
clay and metalsmithing to performance art, and where she began
exploring fabric as an artistic medium. Her MFA thesis was the
Museum School's first performance art thesis. Following her
MFA, she taught at Rhode Island School of Design and Arizona
State University. Cynthia founded the company Transformit in
1987 to produce her architecture and pubic art commission work.
She has taught at Oklahoma Arts Institute, Haystack Mountain
School of Crafts, and lectured at Cranbrook Academy of Art, and
at the Teachers College of Columbia University. Cynthia has
received many awards, including: Art Honors, Maine College of
Art, iF Product Design Award, International Forum Design, Good
Design, Chicago Athenaeum, and twenty-seven consecutive years
of Industrial Fabric Association International notable project
awards. She serves on the board of trustees of Maine College
of Art, and has served on the board of the Maine Coast Waldorf
School, as well as the advisory board for Maine's first creative
economy conference.

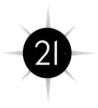

The Great Awareness

Cynthia Thompson

I am an artist. In 1987, I started Transformit, an international company that does artful tension-fabric installations in collaboration with designers and architects. I have always had a lot of energy and rarely sit down. For years, I led a full life that was centered around my daughter, my husband, and my business. Then, everything changed. It was as if I traded in the life I had for a different reality, as if I was swallowed up in a dream world.

It began when I went to Germany on business in January 2011. My company was still struggling from the downturn that shook the economy during the Great Recession. I was not feeling very well. Six months before leaving Germany, I was diagnosed with a urinary tract infection. By the time I left for Germany, the infection had grown worse but I was determined to go because we needed the business.

Two days after arriving in Germany, I ended up in the emergency room. Then I was immediately put in the hospital. I do not speak German and it was a very unnerving situation. I did not get better when they treated me for the urinary tract infection, then they gave me anesthesia to explore what was wrong. I woke up to the doctor telling me that he took out four cancerous tumors in my bladder. It was all like a bad dream: I couldn't believe that he was telling me that I had cancer. Was it really me sitting in that examination room? I couldn't connect to what was happening. It was extremely hard to call home to tell my family that I had cancer. Around this same time, my daughter told me she would be going to college on an art scholarship. I felt joy for her, but I was also scared because she had always been very dependent on me.

My husband Matt immediately came from the United States to take me home. The doctor was caring and straightforward. He said that the cancer got into the bladder wall, which meant that I would have to have my bladder removed. He also said that I should go back to the United States and get three more opinions. As an artist, I visually imagined that I was rotting inside.

The trip back to the United States was tense, since I still did not feel good. When I finally got back I made an appointment with a urologist in Portland, Maine. It was a disaster. At my first appointment, the doctor told me he had already scheduled me for surgery to have my bladder removed. This was *before* he physically examined me, and *before* he saw the pathological slides from Germany. I walked out and started crying and screaming to my husband that I would never go back there. I should have known he was not the doctor for me just from the way his office was decorated, with old surgical tools displayed on the wall; not what an artist wants to see. I quickly proceeded to find another doctor.

I Googled "bladder cancer" and the first place that came up was Massachusetts General Hospital in Boston. The tag line on their Web site said that they save bladders. So off I went to Mass General to meet with a team of doctors. They immediately made me feel safe: they had already read my slides and my C-scan. An added perk was that they bothered to find out who I was as a person by going to my Web site. I was not just a cancer patient to them. It was then that the dream became a reality. They determined that the cancer had not penetrated the bladder wall. So I was scheduled for a biopsy to see for sure. My doctor was Adam Feldman; he had a reassuring manner and looked like a young Gregory Peck. I instinctively trusted him.

The biopsy showed that the cancer had not entered the bladder wall, but that there were still cancer cells present. I then went through six weeks of Bacillus Calmette-Guérin (BCG) treatment. I went to Boston every week and they isolated the treatment to my bladder; after that I had another biopsy, and there were still cancer cells. I went through at least five of these treatments and biopsies, which did not take away the cancer cells. During this time, I started to draw my bladder as a cartoon. It looked like an alien with a smile on its face. I tried to visualize that I would be healthy again. Finally, after I received isolated chemo treatments in my bladder, the biopsy came out negative. (Because the chemo had been localized in my bladder, it did not make me ill or cause my hair to fall out.) After several years, I was now cancer-free.

But the pain of all of the treatments was getting the best of my bladder even though I did not have cancer.

During those treatment years, I did meditation, acupuncture, and exercise, all of which helped but the pain never fully went away. I was urinating at least every fifteen minutes. So I decided to go to the American Biological Center in Scottsdale, Arizona. I found out about this place from the book Dr. *Rau's Swiss Secret.* Along my journey, I read about ten books on cancer and this one made the most sense.

At the center, they put me through a battery of tests that were highly unusual. They tested my energy level and my immune system. Dr. Thom, who was my doctor at the center, said my energy levels and my immune system were at an all-time low, like a glass that was not even half full. Then they gave me treatments of vitamin drips and immune massages (designed to stimulate my immune system), as well as a new diet and supplements. I stayed there a week. Dr. Thom also told me that I should get more sleep and preferably in a dark room.

I had to tell my employees that I would not be around for at least three months. This was a very big thing for me to do. For the next three months almost all I did was sleep. Slowly but surely, I started to get my strength back. My bladder never recovered. It shrunk and did not have the capacity of a healthy bladder. This was starting to have a negative effect on my kidneys so Dr. Feldman, my urologist at Mass General, determined that it was time to remove my bladder even though it was not cancerous. What a blow after three years of doing everything we could to save it.

Luckily, the operation was successful and I do feel better. Before I had the surgery, I went to the American Biological Center and built up my energy so I was in good shape for the operation. I am very grateful to everyone who helped me: Dr. Feldman, Dr. Thom, Dr. Wu, my acupuncturist Mary Chaney, and my meditation therapist Margaret Clements. My husband Matt Rawdon always went to every appointment with me and was by my side to help me through all of the pain. How can I ever thank him? My mom and my daughter also always believed that I would make it. My friends Mark and Sharon generously provided great meals, creative support, and a bed for us in Boston.

So here I am today, working at my company again and doing my art. I still have to remind myself not to get too tired. And also to do the things that get my motor running — Art and Love. The great awareness is: You should always pursue and visualize your "heart's desire." This is what my very good friend Jerry Sanders, performance artist/therapist, taught me. Pursuing your heart's desire will keep you happy and healthy.

JOANNA LAUFER is a writer and editor for a variety of clients. She is the author of *Inspired* (Doubleday) and the co-creator of the best-selling *Inspired* classical music series on RCA. Her nonfiction has appeared in *Child Magazine*, *Dance Spirit*, *Dance Teacher*, *Bottom Line*, and others. Her fiction has appeared in numerous literary journals including *Fiction*, *Ontario Review*, *Antioch Review*, *Greensboro Review*, *StoryQuarterly*, etc. She works privately with authors, editing their manuscripts and readying them for agents and publishers. Joanna is the creator and executive producer of the television series *Dancers: Just Plain Dancing*, and is currently developing scripted and non-scripted television projects.

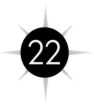

From Nothing to Cancer

Joanna Laufer

The morning the doctor called to say I had cancer, I had been watching a report about salt on the local news. The Board of Health had voted unanimously to require fast-food chains serving high-sodium food to put salt-shaker symbols on their menus. It was a "who cares?" kind of news story, ordinary, like the day. The weather was clear, in the 50s, neither warm nor cold. My husband and I had laughed, as usual, just before he left for the day when our cat tried to block the front door. Just minutes after he left, the telephone rang. I could barely process or believe a word the doctor said. It was like those moments when we note how routine things seemed just before something unfathomable takes place — the beautiful summer day a child drowns, a lovely visit with a friend who is hit by a car the next day.

After that call, nothing seemed ordinary.

219

It was another punch in the gut after a few bad years for my family. My beloved daughter, in her early twenties, had been to three treatment centers for substance abuse. My mother, steadily declining for years, wound up wheelchair-bound with dementia. The day I had my biopsy, she was in the hospital, where she had been for weeks, with an infection that almost killed her. My news, on top of the rest, felt surreal.

About a year before, I had begun spotting, a barely visible, microscopic, faint pink drop of blood. My doctor had reassured me that this was of no concern. I had stopped using suppositories of low-dose estrogen, which were prescribed at the start of menopause. I was told the hormone barely entered the bloodstream and posed no risk. Months later, I read about the risks in every article I Googled. The spotting started happening fairly regularly after sex. My doctor explained that the reason for this was common and simple. Vaginal walls become thin after menopause, hormones help them rebuild, and I had opted not to take them. Why? To lessen my chance of getting cancer.

The change in sex after menopause has been a topic of discussion among my friends. We and our sex drives have had to work around some pain and soreness. We trade recommendations for products that have and haven't helped, like coconut oil, Astroglide, and organic lubricants from a company in England. The majority of my friends didn't have spotting after sex. The ones who did had biopsies immediately. Google this symptom and, despite what any doctor says, articles stress that any bleeding after menopause is suspect. I have always been terrified of medical procedures, and my friends say endometrial biopsies hurt, so I was relieved when I was told I didn't need one.

After a few more weeks of reading articles and feeling anxious, not relieved, I called the doctor and she suggested a sonogram. "I'm not worried at all," she said. "But I know you are." When the doctor saw a polyp in my uterus, I became surprisingly calm. Polyps can cause bleeding, she explained. I was comforted to hear her say she sees them all the time and they are almost always benign.

I never considered myself a candidate for anything other than "benign." I have no family history of uterine cancer. My mother had breast cancer post-menopause and no recurrence for over thirty years. Research claims this significantly lowers the risk of her passing this down to me. I never smoked a cigarette. I exercise daily and eat an extremely healthy diet. I have yearly checkups and seek holistic care. My blood tests and blood pressure are always within the normal range. I never had the flu or a flu shot. I've rarely even had a cold. How could I go from nothing to cancer?

I lived my life believing I had protected myself from this fate. I made healthy choices that allowed me to deceive myself, to push away thoughts of mortality. Pre- and post-diagnosis, I faced two of my greatest fears — surgery and general anesthesia. Never having had either before, I was terrified of so many things; of feeling pain, of being carved up, of being put to death, instead of just put to sleep. And the worst fear of all, the unknown. Would I have cancer? Would it be contained? Would I need chemo or radiation? Would I die?

Here's what not to say to someone pre- or post-diagnosis:

You have to be strong.

You're strong enough to face whatever happens.

Thinking positively can affect the outcome.

It could always be worse.

At your age, you don't need your uterus.

Before the biopsy and the second surgery that removed the cancer, I can't say I felt strong at all. All my prayers and positive thoughts didn't make my polyp benign. There was no comfort in knowing that things could always get worse, that a possible life-threatening disease was now added to the heartbreak over my daughter's addiction and my mother's steady decline. I may not need my uterus and certainly wanted the cancer gone, but there's grief, at any age, when losing part of your body.

Instead say, as my husband said, that you'll be there, that it sucks, that your love is stronger than ever. Discourage searching articles on Google, even if they're true. Ask how it's going and understand that if you hear "fine" it's a lie. Tread lightly if you sense it's a bad time to ask. Offer to visit, as my friends and daughter reassured me they would. Say everything will be okay and be patient if you're asked to repeat it. Enjoy just spending time together, as my mother did, even if you don't know what to do or say.

What did help was a relaxation-before-surgery meditation CD, which I received from the pre-testing nurse at the hospital. I listened to it twice a day. My cat, no matter where he was in the apartment, would come and lay by my lap whenever he heard it playing. The lulling voice guided me to relax every muscle, visualize my favorite peaceful place, and to see myself healed completely. I believe this helped me get through both procedures more easily, with only minimal post-operative pain. What also helped was calling the hospital several times to request that the anesthesiologist angel, who had calmed me and made sure I was spared any side effects during the first operation, would be there again for my second surgery. This took maneuvering since he was one of many and schedules had to be rearranged. At 7:00 a.m., a time-slot I made many phone calls to secure, he was there again helping me through it.

I had to find some way to de-stress, take control, and advocate for myself when so much was out of my hands. I had lost all sense of how to count on good healthy choices, diligence, and luck. I had to fight for my life and composure.

All of this happened a year ago. I don't yet have survival markers that come with Time. I could look back and point to something I could blame — suppositories of estrogen that I was told were safe, not getting a biopsy sooner, my own anxiety that might have contributed to disease. But there's no point in trying to make sense of it. Even things that seem harmless often cause the most harm — air, the sun, Time, Love.

I put all blame aside when I had my first follow-up, knowing the pathology report had come back in my favor. The cancer was contained in the uterus, nowhere else (including nodes), and now, thankfully, it was gone. No further treatment was needed. A male medical student walked into the room before my surgeon arrived. He started explaining, in great detail, about radiation treatment, the manner in which it would be given if my cancer returned. I looked at my husband, who was sitting next to me, a look that let him know I'd had it and that I was alarmed. "Has something changed?" I asked the student. "Do I now need treatment?" "Oh no," he said. "This is just FYI." "Then get out," I said. "Please just get out of here." OUT. Him and cancer.

I have stopped identifying myself as someone who *has* a disease. I look back on it, rather than at it, as something I endured, passed through, made sure I wrapped my voice around by requesting truth, a hint of peace, and speaking up for what I needed. I'm moving on with some caution but mostly with faith. I look to my mother, whose cancer never recurred. I take comfort in this, as a sign of hope, for all of us who had to process and confront unthinkable news, that every fear and challenge we faced will strengthen, heal, and free us.

Singer S Y L V I A M c N A I R , the winner of two Grammy Awards and a Regional Emmy Award, has been on the world's biggest and best stages for thirty-five years, a list that includes the Vienna Philharmonic, the Salzburg Festival, the Metropolitan Opera, the Chicago Symphony, and many more. She has over seventy recordings to her credit ranging from Mozart arias to Brazilian jazz. In May of 2016, her musical autobiography recording, *Subject to Change!*, was released on the Harbinger label. Performances in 2016 include concerts with the Chicago Symphony, the Central City Opera, and A *Robert Shaw Christmas* at the famed Ravinia Festival. Sylvia's true passion lies in the Great American Songbook and in musical theater repertory although her dream of singing on Broadway has yet to be fulfilled and she's not getting any younger! Broadway producers and others are invited to visit Sylvia on Facebook and Twitter.

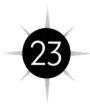

Cancer Is One of the Best Things That Ever Happened to Me

Sylvia McNair

People can't believe it when I say that, but it's true. For me, cancer was more of a cure than a disease. It was the cure for a far worse disease: despair and depression.

My life in music had been rewarding: I had loved singing for and meeting Pope John Paul II at the Vatican (thank you, Vienna Philharmonic) and singing at the Supreme Court (thank you, Justice Sandra Day O'Connor). Then, in early 2006, everything changed. Newly divorced (and unable to even utter the "D" word), changing my career path, with the resulting loss of income and professional stability, feeling like a total failure at everything in life, I sank into a very dark place. I even prayed to die. I believed it couldn't hurt as much as living did.

What do you know, my prayer was answered. In May of 2006, I was diagnosed with an aggressive and advanced breast cancer. "Drop everything and deal with this," one physician said, "NOW!"

The night before my first chemo, I threw a Cancer Party (#1). My closest friends were there along with my physician, my minister, and my attorney.

The following morning, I felt the flow of Adriamycin/ Cytoxan (A/C) go through my right arm and cross my chest, straight to my heart. One poison fighting another. My close friend since third grade, Julie, went to Whole Foods to bring back a healthy lunch — that seemed like a smart thing to do.

The day after A/C infusions, you have to go back to the hospital for Neulasta. Have you seen the price of a shot of Neulasta? Mine was $7,000. Each.

A/C chemo caused my hair to fall out so I threw Cancer Party #2. We ate pizza, drank vodka tonics, and shaved my head.

The summer of 2006 was set to be a very special one. I was scheduled to do one of my dream roles, Mrs. Anna, in my very first production of *The King and I* with

Richard Chamberlain playing the King. Pretty cool! I also had concerts on the books. When the word got out that I was in chemo, every single producer and presenter "dismissed me" but ONE. David Baker. He *insisted* I stay on-board for the Smithsonian Jazz Band concert at the Ravinia Festival in Chicago. So on June 18, 2006, I sang that concert, feeling immensely grateful that David Baker didn't fire me because I had cancer. As if it's contagious . . .

A/C lasted two months until, on July 3, 2006, I was told my tumors were growing while on that hideous cocktail. That was the day I forced the nurse practitioner to tell me the Truth. If I stopped chemo, how long did I have? "Six months," she said, making sure to tell me she didn't like making predictions. I was thankful she broke with professional protocol to tell me the Truth. At least when they tell you the Truth, you have something to work with.

From that appointment, I went directly to the Infusion Lab and . . . sang the National Anthem for everyone! I don't know why I did that. Previously, I had sung the National Anthem in places like Yankee Stadium and

Wrigley Field but that performance on July 3, 2006, in the Infusion Lab at the James Cancer Center of Ohio State University, I remember well.

Surgery #1: Radical Mastectomy. *Take it off, take it off.* Just make sure the nurse who intubates me knows I'm a singer!

My friends threw Cancer Party #3 for me when I got home.

They send you home with these grenade-looking things hanging out of your rib cage. You have to drain them and then measure it every twelve hours. It was weird but nowhere near as weird as what was yet to come three surgeries down the road.

Surgery #2: Port-Catheter Implant. *Veins are shot.*

Three months of Taxotere came next. It was not as bad as A/C but it made me bone-dead tired like nothing I'd ever experienced.

While I was on Taxotere, the ob-gyn I was checking in with did an ultrasound. He saw a lot of things in my uterus that were not supposed to be there. Tumors, cysts, I had them all. He recommended a complete hysterectomy, but to give me a little break, he said we could wait till after I finished Taxotere.

Surgery #3: Eleven days after the last infusion, I had a complete hysterectomy. *Good riddance, menstruation.*

And this is where it gets wild. The recuperation from the hysterectomy went well except for one thing: elimination. All that chemo, three rounds of anesthesia, I figured it was normal. I was wrong. My body had developed more tumors and cysts in my colon and I had a blockage. Several treatments were tried, but none seemed to help. Finally, seventeen days after my hysterectomy, I was forced to undergo an emergency colostomy.

Surgery #4: The Colostomy Bag. This was far-and-away the worst of all. I thought I knew deep, depressing lows but this broke new ground.

Instead of shopping at Nordstrom and Saks that holiday season, I was a regular visitor at the "apparatus store" where I became an expert at bag shapes, adhesives, and deodorizers. I was terrified to be in public. You never know when waste material will pass and it isn't always quiet. I was teaching in a university at the time and the horror I felt of having undergraduates hear or smell this was indescribable.

I went to concerts and the theater but kept my heavy winter coat pressed to my abdomen, hoping it would muffle sound. I sat far away from everyone at church, knowing that "the bag" could make ungodly noises at the most quiet moments. And you can't sleep on your stomach for fear of the damn thing leaking. Waking up to waste material all over yourself is not good.

Medical professionals tried to comfort me by saying things like: "There are thousands of people walking around with permanent colostomies. At least yours is temporary." We hoped.

The *good* news was that the results of both the hysterectomy and the colostomy showed no metastatic disease, no spread of cancer, something that went against every doctor's assumptions.

Thirty-eight sessions of radiation were prescribed. (Really? We can't round it up to forty just to be safe?!) Radiation felt like a vacation compared to the rest of my cancer treatment. My skin handled it with no problems at all and I made sure to impress upon the radiologist that if my vocal cords were, *in any way*, altered by radiation, I would sue her ass off. I didn't really say that but I tried to make the impression that her career had never been on the line quite like it was now.

Surgery #5: Colostomy reversed. The happy ending (pun intended) came in early March 2007, when the most wonderful surgeon in the world stitched me back together . . . and he did it laparoscopically. He works at Indiana University. After ten days in the hospital, I pooped in the toilet, then sent e-mails around the world, announcing it to everyone!

Next, Herceptin. "Just think of it as another protein," a different surgeon told me. So for twelve months, I opened my veins to extra . . . protein.

Then the aromatase inhibitors, Tamoxifen's daughters, the second generation! Chemo by mouth, daily for five years. It was decided I would go on the mighty Arimidex. I didn't tolerate it well and ended up in the ER having *"a heart episode,"* said the adorable ER doc who attended to me that day. My oncologist switched me to Aromasin and I finished out the five years with few problems.

There was a sixth surgery to replace my overworked port with a Power Port so that infusions of contrast dye needed for full-body scans could be more efficiently "pushed" by a machine.

2015: I could not be happier to report that yesterday's blood workup was nothing short of perfect! I am exercising, eating healthy food, teaching, singing all over the place, and enjoying an embarrassingly rich life. I have amazing friendships, a beautiful cocker spaniel who is an angel straight from heaven, and opportunities galore to give back and pay forward, passing along thirty-five years of professional experience to the next generation. Students light my fire. Most importantly, I am grateful for the opportunity to sing my Truth. I consider this the greatest luxury of all: to sing music I love, with people I love, in places I love.

* * *

I started this piece by writing "Cancer Is One of the Best Things That Ever Happened to Me." Here's why:

Cancer forced me to *focus* on the really important questions of life. *Who am I? What do I want? Why do I want it?*

Cancer burns the bullshit out of most of us. Cancer gives us clarity. Cancer showed me I did *not* want to die. I wanted to live! And I wanted to sing everywhere I could!

Cancer cracked my heart open and made it possible for compassion to flow like it had never flowed before.

Nine years have passed since that difficult time in 2006-07 and I would love to say that my commitment to not sweat the small stuff, my promise to be grateful for each day, my desire to remain the better person I was throughout treatment have never wavered. But it's not true. I still battle disappointment and depression. I still get caught in the muck and the mire of work stress. I often don't remember the billions of things I have to be grateful for.

But I don't stay in those wrong-headed places very long. I only have to look at a photograph taken of me the day I came home from the mastectomy, bald as a pool ball, but otherwise looking pretty darn good, to remember the lessons cancer taught me and the *many* gifts it gave me. I wouldn't trade them for anything.

Brooklyn-based P A M E L A R A F A L O W G R O S S M A N has written for outlets such as the *Village Voice*, Time.com, M*s.* magazine, and Salon.com. Her experience with cancer has led her to become a patient's-rights and medical-research advocate, through groups such as the Young Survival Coalition and SHARE. She dedicates this essay in loving memory of her mother, Diana Rafalow Grossman.

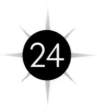

Cancer Island

Pamela Rafalow Grossman

In January of 2008, a doctor who looked about twenty years old — and whom I have never seen since that day — told me I had breast cancer. I was forty years old. I had always been quite healthy; and on top of that, my health habits were somewhat conspicuously squeaky-clean. In high school, friends and I got our hands on cigarettes (of course), but the appeal was lost on me and I ditched them after less than half a pack. In yoga class, my poses were not perfect, but they were heartfelt; I could have been voted "most willing to try." In bars or at parties, I'd nurse a drink or even forget that I had one. A few weeks before my diagnosis, I'd gone hiking in the hills of Los Angeles on almost every day of a vacation and felt just fine.

I think my response to this doctor's news was, "Are you kidding?" She wasn't.

The feeling I had was of suddenly being on an unknown, uncharted island. Everyone else in the room (the doctor, two nurses, and my boyfriend, whose presence I'd firmly requested for whatever this appointment might bring) was on the mainland, where you get to live when you don't have cancer. I had been there, and then, in an instant, I wasn't. I was in this other place; and it had no bridge, no ferry service — no one wanted to make that trip.

I'd been exiled by an unforeseen twist — as my mom and best friend had been by her own cancer diagnosis almost exactly twenty-five years earlier. If my mother had lived, she would of course have helped and advised me through every step of what would come. But she didn't live. As I sat in that small, windowless room, I reminded myself that she is with me every second, in my heart. But beyond that, I could swear I felt her physical presence somewhere near me as I shifted my gaze between the doctor and the floor, blinking back tears.

This Cancer Island is not where anyone wants to be, but one thing to know is that it actually offers great company: Though you feel very alone when you first get there, there are plenty of amazing people navigating its terrain. They, too, feel scared and angry about having ended up there; and they, like you, were in the middle of living full lives before they arrived. They want to talk about and celebrate what means most to them — because a cancer diagnosis may be a part of someone's life, but it does not define that life, and it never will.

I was fortunate to have real love and support around me. I will never forget how I was embraced and surrounded with care. I also found an organization called the Young Survival Coalition, which unites and supports younger women who've been diagnosed with breast cancer. Just as suddenly as I'd been diagnosed, I had a brand-new community available to me.

I have never been much of a big-group person. I'm more of a just-you-and-me planner and an introvert (a chatty introvert, but nonetheless) who chooses friends carefully, one by one. And so I was surprised to find that I quickly adored women all over the country whom I'd never even met in person. I might not have met them, but in chatrooms I read the feelings they expressed about their fears and hopes; their jobs and their sex lives; their decisions about their breasts (lumpectomy or mastectomy? breast reconstruction or none?). Some were married — and hoping their marriages would continue, or even grow stronger, in the face of cancer. Some were dating — and wondering about the protocol for telling a potential partner that, say, one of your breasts is constructed around a silicone implant and has no nipple. Some had children and, of course, wanted fervently to be with them for decades to come. Some didn't have kids and wondered if they still could; or should.

I soaked up all the strength I could get, from my newfound Cancer Island compatriots and my loved ones at large, and tried to reflect it in my approach to cancer treatment. I practiced my Japanese with my Japan-born nurse on my first day of chemo (just a few words, but considering that I was so scared I could hardly speak in any language, not too bad). I began a yoga class for survivors that my yogi friend Lee had recommended. When the time came, I asked my teacher there to cut off my falling-out hair; then I went to a park and threw it into the April grass as bird's-nest material. (I cried the whole time, but still.) I matched my head scarves to my shoes. I joined in a tree-planting project in a park near my home in the middle of chemo, shoveling and dragging wheelbarrows (now, I love to see how the trees have grown since then). Who was that in a blonde wig (my hair is brown) and high heels at a friend's wedding? Right, me.

In the almost nine years since my diagnosis, I've seen countless triumphs within my young-survivor community. Promotions and pregnancies; engagements and the buying of homes; businesses and not-for-profits launched; adoptions joyfully announced. For us, milestones that others take for granted can be cause for celebration. Women who dreamed of seeing a child start kindergarten are thrilled to watch that preteen begin middle school. Getting approved to buy life insurance is a very big deal.

Something I've learned over these years is that even if I remain cancer-free and live to be 102, which is the plan, some part of me will always be on Cancer Island. On some days it's a toe, on some days a foot; on some days — for example, when I lose one of my friends to cancer — it's most of me. I will never again be 100 percent not there. I'll take this opportunity to apologize to anyone who has tried to tell me something during the years since my diagnosis and been met with a faraway stare. Sometimes the news in this community is not good. Sometimes someone I love is struggling mightily, receiving word that what had been a highly successful treatment is now failing to work at all. At those times, it's hard for me to think of anything else.

So — Cancer Island will remain a part of me, my citizenship there always current; I will travel back and forth between it and the rest of my life. In some ways that's a heavy burden; but in other ways it isn't. My will is stronger as a result. My bullshit meter is much more finely tuned. I give myself time to address what's most important; and the things that don't matter *really* don't matter to me now. (I still catch myself stressing over them sometimes, but it's much easier to break that cycle.) I used to beat myself up for any and every mistake; now I make a point of reflecting on my successes as well. I used to feel lazy if I let myself have a lunch break; now I know that I'm allowed, as are we all, and that if at all possible, I should take a few minutes to breathe fresh air in the middle of the day.

I was always a dedicated celebrator of friends' birthdays and my own, but now my enthusiasm has been turned up a few notches. This is partly in honor of the many incredible people out there with Stage IV cancer, who do everything they can to reach their next birthday celebration. If invited, I will most likely attend your birthday party, with gusto. Hell, I will help plan your birthday party. The loudest voice in the crowd singing "Happy birthday" will often be mine.

Cancer and cancer treatment have been, I can't lie, hard on my body; and sometimes that in itself makes me very sad. My options for creating a family are still a work in progress, when I'd hoped that issue would have been settled a while back. Recurrence-prevention drugs that affect my hormones accordingly affect everything from my hair to my weight to my ability to retrieve, with my previous speed, the word I'm looking for. (I also read — and have unsuccessfully tried to forget — that chemo alone can age the body by about ten years.) But my relationship with Cancer Island has strengthened my spirit, and how can I be sorry about that?

Here's to all of us, whichever islands of life we find ourselves on — growing and reaching, building bridges, using our strength to its best purposes, for all the decades after.

JOAN LUNDEN was the cohost of *Good Morning America* for nearly two decades, bringing insight to the day's top stories, from presidential elections to issues of health and wellness. Her best-selling books include *Joan Lunden's Healthy Cooking*, *Joan Lunden's Healthy Living*, *Wake-Up Calls*, and *A Bend in the Road Is Not the End of the Road*. Joan speaks all over the country about health and wellness, inspiration, and success. Her Web site, JoanLunden.com, and her social media have quickly become go-to destinations for information and support within the breast cancer community, bringing together experts on a myriad of relevant topics for today's woman. In October 2014, Joan joined NBC's *Today Show* as a Special Correspondent for Breast Cancer Awareness Month.

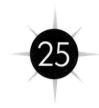

Had I Known

Joan Lunden
with Laura Morton

It's time to wake up!

We need early screening and, when necessary, ancillary screenings to be made available to every woman and covered by insurance.

Just consider the facts: We are seeing more and more women in their twenties, thirties, and certainly forties being diagnosed with breast cancer, and researchers are frantically trying to figure out why.

Doesn't this clearly show that early screening is more critical than ever?

As much as this cancer has tried to beat me down, somehow it has also grown me a big ol' set of balls. I'll be careful not to wear my skirts too short when I go to Washington to advocate, so they won't show. But as long as I grew them, I might as well use them.

There's no question that we've made great strides in our fight against breast cancer, but my experience, combined with those of so many other women diagnosed with the disease, shows that we still have a lot of work to do. Many people have worked tirelessly to raise awareness, to spread the word that breast cancer is a threat to women everywhere, and to suggest that funds are needed for more research. As a result, we have achieved great awareness around the country about breast cancer.

When the NFL is wearing pink during October, I think we've got plenty of awareness.

What I believe we need more of now is *education*.

Thankfully, millions of women are now receiving routine mammograms, but going forward, I hope that we shift the focus to better tailor health-care screenings to fit each woman's individual needs. *Breast cancer care cannot be one-size-fits-all.*

It is a very heterogeneous disease. It is a cancer that I believe requires great personalization. What's right for one woman isn't necessarily right for another, and approaching it as a one-size-fits-all issue undermines the true abilities that we have to combat breast cancer.

I hope there will be a day when we can get gynecologists and other referring doctors to discuss the issue of breast density with their female patients. Women have been kept in the dark on this issue far too long.

Had I known that my radiologist had been giving lifesaving information to my gynecologist for decades that wasn't being passed on to me, I would have been able to have an intelligent conversation about my risk factors. Instead, I stuck my head in the sand, thinking and believing that because I didn't have a family history of breast cancer, I was somehow immune.

Had I known that dense breast tissue increases your risk of cancer, maybe I would have been more vigilant in my care. I hope that as we go forward, we'll focus research not only on treatment but on *prevention* and which lifestyle factors and habits might alter breast cancer risk and recurrence — exercise, weight, diet, and stress.

Had I known how bad sugar is for you — that it is like jet fuel for the growth of cancer cells — hello,

I would have cut it out of my diet a long time ago. It's sugar's relationship to higher insulin levels and related growth factors that may influence cancer cell growth the most.

And I don't even have a sweet tooth! In fact, I couldn't care less about desserts. But *had I known* just how dangerous it was, I never would have succumbed to a warm chocolate chip cookie or a hot fudge sundae on that cross-country flight, which was where I usually indulged, because I am not a dessert eater. Admittedly, it's hard to say no when they bake those cookies in the galley and the entire cabin fills with the sweet smell of freshly baked chocolate chip cookies. There's something comforting about it that teases the brain into saying yes when you ought to say no.

Willpower be damned!

Sometimes when the flight attendant came by with that silver tray, I closed my eyes tight, stuck my fingers in my ears, and sang "la-la-la-la-la" until she got the idea and tempted the next passenger with her dessert.

Had I known my life was actually in danger, it would have been so easy just to say no.

And now that I know, I cannot unlearn all of this.

But I can and will pass it along.

Going forward, I will share with others what I've learned about the signals that foods can send to your cells, how some foods put you at risk and others actually protect you.

I hope that as we go forward, doctors won't recommend the same treatment to every woman, just because that's the way it's always been done, if there is something new and more promising that better fits her particular needs. This is a field where research discoveries change detection, treatment, and survival rates week to week, month to month.

I think I'm a good example that trying a new regimen brought a good outcome.

I hope that as we go forward, we focus on treating the whole woman and not just the cancer.

I hope that doctors consider the long-term side effects that can result from the cancer treatment itself. It's easy for doctors and patients to focus on the more immediate and obvious side effects — like hair loss from chemo — and those unfortunately can and often do trump discussion about the long-term side effects that may occur after chemotherapy.

Finally, I hope that as we go forward, we can *focus on the doctor-patient relationship*. I am aware that I had the very best medical care available. I had it so good. However, in going public with my cancer journey and connecting with thousands of women who have shared their stories, I am also aware that not everyone has had the same quality care.

I was extremely fortunate to have incredibly wonderful relationships with my doctors. Each one helped me to understand my disease and all of the treatment options available to me.

I am making a promise here and now.

I will look for every opportunity to put myself in front of medical professionals and impress upon them the importance of their relationship with you and what you need from them:

1. To always share pertinent lifesaving information;

2. To probe and help you ascertain what your real risk factors for cancer may be;

3. To see that you get any and all ancillary tests that may be required, considering your health circumstances;

4. To explain all of the potential treatment paths available and why certain ones may better fit your needs;

5. To communicate with all other doctors treating you so that you get the best care; and

6. To remember that other, very important prescription: a caring and comforting smile and a word of encouragement that together we can beat this, and that you must stay positive and believe you can beat this, and that you may or may not have some lousy days, but in the end, you will survive!

About the Editor

Mark Evan Chimsky is the head of Mark Chimsky Editorial Services Unlimited, an editorial consulting business based in Portland, Maine. For nearly six years, he was the editor in chief of the book division of Sellers Publishing, an independent publishing company in South Portland, Maine. Previously he was executive editor and editorial director of Harper San Francisco and headed the paperback divisions at Little, Brown and Macmillan. In addition, he was on the faculty of New York University's Center for Publishing, and for three years he served as the director of the book section of NYU's Summer Publishing Institute. He has edited a number of best-selling books, including Johnny Cash's memoir, Cash, and he has worked with such notable authors as Melody Beattie, Arthur Hertzberg, Beryl Bender Birch, and Robert Coles. He was also project manager on Billy Graham's New York Times best-selling memoir, Just As I Am. He conceived of the long-running series The Best American Erotica, which was compiled by Susie Bright, and he was the first editor to reissue the works of celebrated novelist Dawn Powell. His editorial achievements have been noted in Vanity Fair, the Nation, and Publishers Weekly. He is an award-winning poet whose poetry and essays have appeared in JAMA (the Journal of the American Medical Association), Wild Violet, Three Rivers Poetry Journal, and Mississippi Review. For Sellers Publishing, he developed and compiled a number of acclaimed books, including Creating a Life You'll Love, which won the silver in ForeWord's 2009 Book of the Year Awards (self-help category) and 65 Things to Do When You Retire, which the Wall Street Journal called "[one of] the year's best guides to later life." In addition to helping authors develop marketable proposals and manuscripts, Mark teaches in the Writing, Literature, and Publishing Department at Emerson College in Boston.

Acknowledgments

Books always start with the spark of an idea. In this case, that spark came from Ronnie Sellers, President and Publisher of Sellers Publishing, and I want to express my deep thanks to him for trusting me with his vision for this book. His feedback, support, and advocacy are greatly appreciated.

This book is as uplifting as it is because of all the women who contributed to it. They agreed to share their stories of pain and hope in an effort to help others, and the experience of working with them was truly inspiring. In addition to their candor and courage, their generosity extended to providing their essays free of charge since all royalties from the sale of the book will be donated to nonprofits dedicated to cancer research and prevention.

The process of putting this book together was enriched by a number of people behind the scenes who provided invaluable assistance along the way. They include Cristina Abaroa, Nava Atlas, Frederick Courtright, Lucy Davis, Alicia Dercole, Shaun Dreisbach, Cindy Hounsell, Lindsay Krauss Weinberg, Katie Leighton, Dorian Mintzer, Erica Moroz, Lisa Perkins, Chris Staros, and Matt Yorio.

I also want to thank the wonderful staff at Sellers Publishing, particularly Mary Baldwin, Charlotte Cromwell, and Sue Wight for making this book look as good as it does; and to Megan Hiller for her expert proofreading.

Last but not least, I want to acknowledge Robin Haywood, Laurie Moore Skillings, Kimberly Gladman, and Joanna Laufer, who gave me their wise counsel and encouragement throughout the long process of researching, compiling, and editing this project. I am grateful to them for the gift of their sustaining friendship as they joined me on this extraordinary journey.

Credits